**BMA**

# SBAs, EMQs & SAQs in
# MEDICINE

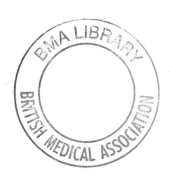
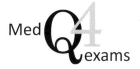
Med Q4 exams

tfm Publishing Limited, Castle Hill Barns, Harley, Shrewsbury, SY5 6LX, UK
Tel: +44 (0)1952 510061; Fax: +44 (0)1952 510192
E-mail: info@tfmpublishing.com; Web site: www.tfmpublishing.com

Editing, design & typesetting: Nikki Bramhill BSc Hons Dip Law
Cover photo: © iStock.com
Success smart medical doctor working with operating room as concept (Pablo_K) —
Stock photo ID: 629432686

| First edition: | © 2019 |
| Paperback | ISBN: 978-1-910079-71-3 |
| E-book editions: | © 2019 |
| ePub | ISBN: 978-1-910079-72-0 |
| Mobi | ISBN: 978-1-910079-73-7 |
| Web pdf | ISBN: 978-1-910079-74-4 |

Printed by Gutenberg Press Ltd., Gudja Road, Tarxien, GXQ 2902, Malta
Tel: +356 2398 2201; Fax: +356 2398 2290
E-mail: info@gutenberg.com.mt; Web site: www.gutenberg.com.mt

# Contents

# About the Editor

Dr. Matthew Hanks graduated from the University of Sheffield in 2015 with an MBChB in medicine; prior to this Matthew studied for a BSc Biomedical Science degree in Sheffield graduating in 2010 with a first class honours degree. He has a keen interest in teaching and has devised many different teaching programmes for students which have been engaging and received positive feedback. He now hopes to take this passion further by providing students with resources that are both useful and informative to enhance their learning opportunities.

# Contributors

**Dr. Gemma Adams MBChB**
Clinical Fellow in General Medicine and Geriatrics, South Yorkshire Deanery

**Dr. Paul Galaway BA MBBS MRCP**
CT2 Core Medical Trainee, Yorkshire and The Humber Deanery

**Dr. Vanessa Halford BSc (Hons) MBChB MRCP**
CT2 Core Medical Trainee, Yorkshire and The Humber Deanery

**Dr. Matthew Hanks BSc (Hons) MBChB PG Cert Surgery**
CT2 Core Surgical Trainee, East Midlands North Deanery

**Dr. Richard Harrold MBChB (Hons)**
Locum Senior House Officer, South Yorkshire Region

**Dr. Amelia Lloyd BMedSci MBChB**
F2 Sandwell and West Birmingham Hospitals NHS Trust

**Dr. Rebecca Marlor BMedSci (Hons) MBChB**
CT2 Core Medical Trainee, Yorkshire and The Humber Deanery

**Dr. Morwenna Read BMedSci (Hons) MBChB (Hons)**
F2 Sheffield Teaching Hospitals NHS Foundation Trust

**Dr. Emily Reed BMedSci MBChB**
F2 Sheffield Teaching Hospitals NHS Foundation Trust

# Acknowledgements

I would like to thank all those who have taken the time to contribute to this title which is the amalgamation of knowledge from professionals studying and working all over the United Kingdom; without their hard work and dedication, this book would not have been possible.

Mrs Maxine Ward and Mrs Lisa Wheatley have been instrumental in locating many of the ECGs found throughout this book and without their commitment and enthusiasm the clear examples of common ECG findings in a variety of conditions found in this publication would not have been possible.

I would also like to thank Megan Ward and Glenda Hanks for their patience whilst the book has developed and for the support of Nikki Bramhill from tfm Publishing who has guided me through the many hurdles of publishing.

Matthew Hanks
June 2019

# Normal reference values

Please note normal reference values may vary between different hospitals.

| | |
|---|---|
| Hb | Male 131-166g/L |
| | Female 110-147g/L |
| MCV | 81-96fL |
| Platelets | 150-400 x $10^9$/L |
| WCC | 3.5-9.5 x $10^9$/L |
| Neutrophils | 1.7-6.5 x $10^9$/L |
| Lymphocytes | 1.0-3.0 x $10^9$/L |
| Eosinophils | 0.04-0.5 x $10^9$/L |
| Basophils | 0.0-0.25 x $10^9$/L |
| Sodium | 133-146mmol/L |
| Potassium | 3.5-5.3mmol/L |
| Urea | 2.5-7.8mmol/L |
| Creatinine | 62-106µmol/L |
| eGFR | >90 |
| | |
| Calcium | 2.25-2.5mmol/L |
| | |
| Total protein | 60-80g/L |
| Globulin | 18-36g/L |
| Bilirubin | 0-21µmol/L |
| ALT | 0-41iU/L |
| ALP | 30-130iU/L |

| | |
|---|---|
| AST | 0-35iU/L |
| Albumin | 35-50g/L |
| | |
| PT | 10.1-11.8 seconds |
| APTT | 20.2-28.7 seconds |
| Thrombin time | 11.3-17.4 seconds |
| Fibrinogen | 2.0-4.0g/L |
| | |
| CRP | 0-5mg/L |

# Abbreviations

| | |
|---|---|
| AAA | Abdominal aortic aneurysm |
| ABG | Arterial blood gas |
| ACE | Angiotensin-converting enzyme |
| ACTH | Adrenocorticotrophic hormone |
| ADH | Antidiuretic hormone |
| AF | Atrial fibrillation |
| AIDS | Acquired immunodeficiency syndrome |
| AKI | Acute kidney injury |
| ALL | Acute lymphoblastic leukaemia |
| ALP | Alkaline phosphatase |
| ALS | Advanced Life Support |
| ALT | Alanine aminotransferase |
| AML | Acute myeloid leukaemia |
| ANA | Anti-nuclear antibodies |
| ANCA | Anti-neutrophil cytoplasmic antibodies |
| APTT | Activated partial thromboplastin time |
| ARDS | Adult respiratory distress syndrome |
| ASA | American Society of Anesthesiologists |
| AST | Aspartate aminotransferase |
| ATP | Adenosine triphosphate |
| AV | Atrioventricular |
| AVM | Arteriovenous malformation |
| BBV | Blood-borne virus |
| BMI | Body Mass Index |
| BP | Blood pressure |
| BPM | Beats per minute |
| CA19-9 | Carbohydrate antigen 19-9 |

| | |
|---|---|
| CAH | Congenital adrenal hyperplasia |
| CBT | Cognitive behavioural therapy |
| CCF | Congestive cardiac failure |
| CJD | Creutzfeldt-Jakob disease |
| CK | Creatinine kinase |
| CKD | Chronic kidney disease |
| Cl⁻ | Chloride |
| CLO | *Campylobacter*-like organism |
| CML | Chronic myeloid leukaemia |
| CNS | Central nervous system |
| COPD | Chronic obstructive pulmonary disease |
| CPAP | Continuous positive airway pressure |
| CRP | C-reactive protein |
| CSF | Cerebrospinal fluid |
| CT | Computed tomography |
| CTPA | Computed tomography pulmonary angiography |
| CXR | Chest X-ray |
| DC | Direct current |
| DEXA | Dual energy X-ray absorptiometry |
| DI | Diabetes insipidus |
| DIC | Disseminated intravascular coagulation |
| DIP | Distal interphalangeal joint |
| DKA | Diabetic ketoacidosis |
| DMARD | Disease modifying anti-rheumatic drug |
| DOAC | Direct-acting oral anticoagulant |
| DPP-4 | Dipeptidyl peptidase-4 |
| DVT | Deep vein thrombosis |
| EBV | Epstein-Barr virus |
| ECG | Electrocardiogram |
| EEG | Electroencephalogram |
| ESR | Erythrocyte sedimentation rate |
| FBC | Full blood count |
| FiO$_2$ | Fraction of inspired oxygen |

| | |
|---|---|
| G6PD | Glucose-6-phosphate dehydrogenase |
| GBM | Glomerular basement membrane |
| GCA | Giant cell arteritis |
| GCS | Glasgow Coma Scale |
| GFR | Glomerular filtration rate |
| GH | Growth hormone |
| GI | Gastrointestinal |
| GORD | Gastro-oesophageal reflux disease |
| GTN | Glyceryl trinitrate |
| $H^+$ | Hydrogen |
| HADS | Hospital Anxiety and Depression Scale |
| HAV | Hepatitis A virus |
| Hb | Haemoglobin |
| HBcAB | Hepatitis B core antibody |
| HBcAg | Hepatitis B core antigen |
| HbeAB | Hepatitis B e antibody |
| HBeAg | Hepatitis B e antigen |
| HBsAB | Hepatitis B surface antibody |
| HBsAg | Hepatitis B surface antigen |
| HBV | Hepatitis B virus |
| HDV | Hepatitis D virus |
| HEV | Hepatitis E virus |
| HHS | Hyperosmolar hyperglycaemic state |
| HIV | Human immunodeficiency virus |
| HLA | Human leucocyte antigen |
| HPV | Human papilloma virus |
| HRT | Hormone replacement therapy |
| HSP | Henoch-Schönlein purpura |
| HSV | Herpes simplex virus |
| HZV | Herpes zoster virus |
| IBD | Inflammatory bowel disease |
| IBS | Irritable bowel syndrome |
| Ig | Immunoglobulin |

| | |
|---|---|
| IM | Intramuscular |
| INR | International Normalised Ratio |
| ITP | Idiopathic thrombocytopenic purpura |
| IV | Intravenous |
| JVP | Jugular venous pressure |
| K⁺ | Potassium |
| LDH | Lactate dehydrogenase |
| LFT | Liver function test |
| LMWH | Low-molecular-weight heparin |
| LRTI | Lower respiratory tract infection |
| MCA | Middle cerebral artery |
| MC&S | Microscopy, culture and sensitivity |
| MCP | Metacarpophalangeal joint |
| MCV | Mean corpuscular volume |
| MEN | Multiple endocrine neoplasia |
| MGUS | Monoclonal gammopathy of undetermined significance |
| MI | Myocardial infarction |
| MMSE | Mini-mental state examination |
| MND | Motor neurone disease |
| MRI | Magnetic resonance imaging |
| MRSA | Methicillin-resistant *Staphylococcus aureus* |
| MS | Multiple sclerosis |
| MTP | Metatarsophalangeal joint |
| MuSK | Muscle specific kinase |
| MUST | Malnutrition Universal Screening Tool |
| Na⁺ | Sodium |
| NG | Nasogastric |
| NJ | Nasojejunal |
| NMDA | N-methyl-D-aspartate |
| NSAID | Non-steroidal anti-inflammatory drug |
| NSTEMI | Non-ST elevation myocardial infarction |
| NYHA | New York Heart Association |
| OD | Once daily |

| | |
|---|---|
| OGD | Oesophagogastroduodenoscopy |
| PAS | Periodic acid-Schiff |
| PBC | Primary biliary cirrhosis |
| PE | Pulmonary embolism |
| PEFR | Peak expiratory flow rate |
| PEG | Percutaneous endoscopic gastrostomy |
| PEJ | Percutaneous endoscopic jejunostomy |
| PERC | Pulmonary embolism rule out criteria |
| PHQ-9 | Patient Health Questionnaire-9 |
| PIP | Proximal interphalangeal joint |
| PO | *Per os* (oral administration) |
| PPI | Proton pump inhibitor |
| PRV | Polycythaemia rubra vera |
| PSC | Primary sclerosing cholangitis |
| PT | Prothrombin time |
| PTH | Parathyroid hormone |
| RBC | Red blood cell |
| SIADH | Syndrome of inappropriate antidiuretic hormone |
| SIRS | Systemic inflammatory response syndrome |
| SLE | Systemic lupus erythematosus |
| SSRI | Selective serotonin reuptake inhibitor |
| STEMI | ST-elevation myocardial infarction |
| SVC | Superior vena cava |
| T3 | Tri-iodothyronine |
| T4 | Thyroxine |
| TB | Tuberculosis |
| TDS | *Ter die sumendum* (three times a day) |
| TIA | Transient ischaemic attack |
| TNF | Tumour necrosis factor |
| TPN | Total parenteral nutrition |
| TSH | Thyroid-stimulating hormone |
| tTG | Tissue transglutaminase antibodies |
| U&Es | Urea & electrolytes |

| | |
|---|---|
| URTI | Upper respiratory tract infection |
| USS | Ultrasound scan |
| UTI | Urinary tract infection |
| VBG | Venous blood gas |
| VF | Ventricular fibrillation |
| V/Q | Ventilation/perfusion ratio |
| VTE | Venous thromboembolism |
| vWF | von Willebrand factor |
| WBC | White blood cell |
| WCC | White cell count |
| $\gamma$-GT | Gamma-glutamyl transferase |

# Section 1
# Questions

# Chapter 1

# Cardiology
## QUESTIONS

## Single best answer questions

1) A 30-year-old female presents with palpitations and is found to have regular, narrow complex tachycardia. Vagal manoeuvres and adenosine 6mg IV fail to resolve the tachyarrhythmia. What is the next most appropriate step?

a. Adenosine 6mg IV.
b. Adenosine 12mg IV.
c. Verapamil 5mg IV.
d. Amiodarone 600mg IV loading dose.

2) A 65-year-old male is receiving treatment for infective endocarditis when he suddenly develops pruritis and an erythematous rash over his face, neck and torso during a vancomycin infusion. What is the most appropriate step?

a. Stop the infusion.
b. Pause the infusion and reset at a slower rate.
c. Give chlorphenamine.
d. Give hydrocortisone.

3) A 70-year-old female develops severe community-acquired pneumonia for which she is prescribed co-amoxiclav and clarithromycin. Which of the following medications should be withheld?

a. Atorvastatin.
b. Ramipril.
c. Bisoprolol.
d. Isosorbide mononitrate.

4) A 65-year-old male with known angina presents to the emergency department in AF with bothersome palpitations. He develops complete heart block following the administration of which medication?

a. Adenosine.
b. Amiodarone.
c. Bisoprolol.
d. Ivabradine.

5) A 43-year-old presents to the clinic for a routine follow-up for hypertrophic cardiomyopathy. What character of pulse is most likely to be felt?

a) Bisferens.
b) Collapsing.
c) Jerky.
d) Slow rising.

6) A patient is diagnosed with congestive cardiac failure. Which of the following medications provides a prognostic benefit?

a. Bumetanide.
b. Digoxin.
c. Furosemide.
d. Ramipril.

7) A patient of Afro-Caribbean origin is referred to the hypertension clinic with an ambulatory blood pressure recording of 165/100mmHg. What is the most appropriate management?

a. Amlodipine.
b. Hydralazine.
c. Lifestyle advice.
d. Ramipril.

8) Which of the following carries the worst prognosis in symptomatic aortic stenosis?

a. Angina.
b. Exertional syncope.
c. Slow rising pulse.
d. Shortness of breath.

9) A 42-year-old male presents to his primary care doctor with a 5-day history of shortness of breath, fatigue and ankle swelling. On examination, a pansystolic murmur is detected loudest at the left fifth intercostal space in the mid-clavicular line radiating to the axilla. What is the most likely diagnosis?

a. Aortic stenosis.
b. Tricuspid regurgitation.
c. Mitral regurgitation.
d. Mitral stenosis.

10) A 56-year-old male develops crushing chest pain with ST changes consistent with ST-elevation myocardial infarction. To where is radiation of pain most specific for acute myocardial infarction?

a.   Left shoulder.
b.   Back.
c.   Right shoulder.
d.   Right thorax.

11) A previously fit and well 53-year-old female is diagnosed with non-ST elevation myocardial infarction. Which two medications must be prescribed before proceeding to primary percutaneous intervention?

a.   Aspirin and glyceryl trinitrate spray.
b.   Aspirin and ticagrelor.
c.   Bisoprolol and glyceryl trinitrate spray.
d.   Ramipril and bisoprolol.

12) Following an ST-elevation myocardial infarction, a patient develops shortness of breath and an echocardiograph demonstrates severe left ventricular impairment. The patient is currently taking aspirin, ticagrelor, ramipril, atorvastatin and bisoprolol. Which medication is indicated as an adjunct to the current medical therapy?

a.   Digoxin.
b.   Eplerenone.
c.   Furosemide.
d.   Spironolactone.

13) Which of the following is not a sign or symptom of left-sided heart failure?

a. Ankle swelling.
b. Fatigue.
c. Shortness of breath.
d. Tachycardia.

14) Following a myocardial infarction, a patient develops a cough. Current medication includes: aspirin, ticagrelor, atorvastatin, bisoprolol, ramipril and glyceryl trinitrate. On examination, there is no peripheral oedema and good air entry bilaterally. What is the next most appropriate management step?

a. Start digoxin.
b. Start furosemide.
c. Stop ramipril and start losartan.
d. Stop ticagrelor and start clopidogrel.

15) A 64-year-old female presents with severe, crushing chest pain and an ECG demonstrates ventricular tachycardia. What is the most appropriate management?

a. Amiodarone 300mg IV followed by 900mg over 24 hours.
b. DC cardioversion.
c. Metoprolol 5mg IV.
d. Verapamil 5mg IV.

16) A 45-year-old female is diagnosed with a non-ST elevation myocardial infarction and chooses medical therapy. When can the patient recommence driving a car?

a. Seventy-two hours.
b. One week.
c. Four weeks.
d. Six months.

17) A 56-year-old male undergoes a percutaneous coronary intervention following a non-ST elevation myocardial infarction and has an uneventful recovery. When can he recommence driving a car or motorcycle?

a. Seventy-two hours.
b. One week.
c. Four weeks.
d. Six months.

18) A 50-year-old Caucasian male attends his primary care doctor for a routine check-up. His blood pressure is elevated at 148/94mmHg. It has been persistently raised over the past 18 months in clinic and using ambulatory home blood pressure monitoring. What would be the first-line treatment offered to this patient?

a. Amiloride.
b. Amlodipine.
c. Hydralazine.
d. Ramipril.

19) A patient presents with severe headaches after starting a new medication for their angina. This is a common side effect of which of the following medications?

a.  Bisoprolol.
b.  Digoxin.
c.  Isosorbide mononitrate.
d.  Ivabradine.

20) A 20-year-old male was found collapsed on the street. An ECG was performed. What does this ECG show?

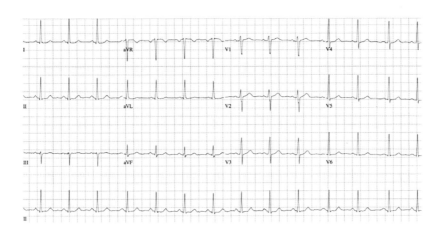

a.  Atrial ectopic beats.
b.  Normal sinus rhythm.
c.  Atrial fibrillation.
d.  Wolff-Parkinson-White syndrome.

21) A 55-year-old female is admitted to the emergency department following a collapse. The ambulance crew have provided you with an ECG obtained at the scene. What does this ECG show?

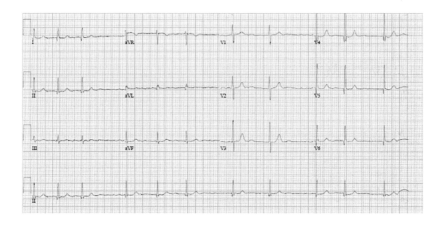

a. Atrial fibrillation.
b. Second-degree heart block, Mobitz Type I.
c. Second-degree heart block, Mobitz Type II.
d. Third-degree heart block.

22) A patient presents with crushing chest pain. An ECG is performed in the emergency department. What does this ECG suggest?

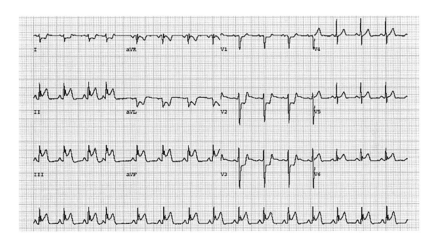

a.   Anterior NSTEMI.
b.   Anterior STEMI.
c.   Inferior STEMI.
d.   Pericarditis.

23) A 42-year-old female presents to the emergency department with a 4-hour history of chest pain and shortness of breath. She recently underwent a mastectomy. An ECG is performed. What is the most likely diagnosis?

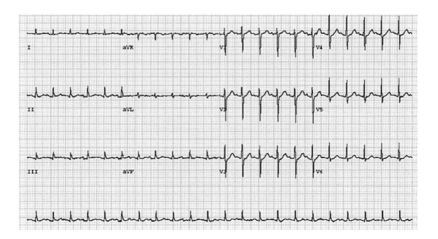

a.   Pericarditis.
b.   Pulmonary embolism.
c.   Anterior STEMI.
d.   Wolff-Parkinson-White syndrome.

# Extended matching questions

## Characteristic signs on examination

a.  Bisferens pulse.                 e.  Tapping apex beat.
b.  Jerky pulse.                     f.  Corrigan's sign.
c.  Slow rising pulse.               g.  De Musset's sign.
d.  Collapsing pulse.                h.  Pulsus paradoxus.

## Match the sign to the underlying diagnosis.

1) Cardiac tamponade.

2) Aortic stenosis.

3) Mixed aortic stenosis and aortic regurgitation.

4) Mitral stenosis.

5) Hypertrophic obstructive cardiomyopathy.

## Congestive cardiac failure functional status

| | | | |
|---|---|---|---|
| a. | NYHA Class I. | e. | ASA I. |
| b. | NYHA Class II. | f. | ASA II. |
| c. | NYHA Class III. | g. | ASA III. |
| d. | NYHA Class IV. | h. | ASA IV. |

Identify the functional status of the following patients with congestive cardiac failure below.

6) No limitations to activity.

7) A patient has a difficulty breathing and feels profoundly tired at rest.

8) A patient is unable to run upstairs due to weakness and breathlessness, but is unlimited on flat ground.

9) A patient is comfortable at rest, but becomes short of breath on minimal exertion.

10) Following insertion of a cardiac resynchronisation device, a largely bed-bound patient was able to mobilise independently with a walking stick.

## Medication side effects

a. Digoxin.
b. Adenosine.
c. Ramipril.
d. Spironolactone.

e. Furosemide.
f. Bendroflumethiazide.
g. Amiodarone.
h. Aspirin.

Match the medication with the common side effect below.

11) A sense of impending doom.

12) Tinnitus.

13) Slate-coloured skin.

14) Gastritis.

15) Bothersome cough.

## Complications of acute myocardial infarction

| | | | |
|---|---|---|---|
| a. | Complete heart block. | e. | Congestive cardiac failure. |
| b. | Pericarditis. | f. | Cardiac tamponade. |
| c. | Dressler's syndrome. | g. | Mural thrombus. |
| d. | Ventricular aneurysm. | h. | Mitral regurgitation. |

Match the sequela from myocardial infarction with the presentation.

16) A patient presents with pleuritic chest pain relieved by leaning forward following an acute MI.

17) A patient presents with their third episode of ventricular tachycardia and evidence of left-sided heart failure 4 weeks following an MI.

18) A patient develops profound left-sided weakness following an MI.

19) A patient develops flash pulmonary oedema and a new systolic murmur following an MI.

20) An 80-year-old gentleman presents to his primary care doctor with sharp chest pain 3 days following an episode of crushing chest pain.

## Management of hypertension

| | | | |
|---|---|---|---|
| a. | Amlodipine. | e. | Verapamil. |
| b. | Labetalol. | f. | Ivabradine. |
| c. | Bendroflumethiazide. | g. | Ramipril. |
| d. | Indapamide. | h. | Losartan. |

Select the next most appropriate medication for the clinic scenario.

21) White Caucasian aged 60 years with a first presentation of hypertension (BP 170/95mmHg on an ambulatory blood pressure monitor).

22) A 65-year-old male currently on amlodipine 10mg with a blood pressure consistently greater than 160mmHg systolic and 100mmHg diastolic.

23) A patient on maximum doses of amlodipine and ramipril and has a consistently elevated systolic blood pressure of >170mmHg.

24) A 30-year-old female with gestational diabetes with a blood pressure of 150/105mmHg.

25) A 35-year-old male of Afro-Caribbean origin presents with a persistently elevated systolic blood pressure of >180mmHg.

## Cardiac sounds

a.  Aortic stenosis.                    e.  Tricuspid regurgitation.
b.  Aortic regurgitation.               f.  Tricuspid stenosis.
c.  Mitral stenosis.                    g.  Pulmonary stenosis.
d.  Mitral regurgitation.               h.  Pulmonary regurgitation.

## Match the diagnosis to the clinical sign.

26) Loud first heart sound and diastolic murmur.

27) Pansystolic murmur enhanced on expiration.

28) Ejection systolic murmur with radiation to carotids.

29) Pansystolic murmur enhanced on inspiration.

30) High-pitched diastolic murmur with an S3 heart sound best heard at
    the left sternal border.

## Tachycardia

| | | | |
|---|---|---|---|
| a. | DC cardioversion. | e. | Valsalva manoeuvres. |
| b. | Verapamil. | f. | Amiodarone. |
| c. | Metoprolol. | g. | Magnesium sulphate. |
| d. | Adenosine. | h. | Ivabradine. |

Match the arrhythmia with the most appropriate treatment.

31) A patient presents with palpitation. The ECG demonstrates ventricular tachycardia. There is no haemodynamic compromise or chest pain.

32) A patient presents with dizziness. Persistent AF occurs on ECGs over 2 days. The past medical history includes brittle asthma and Type 2 diabetes.

33) A patient presents with dizziness. The ECG shows a regular narrow complex tachycardia.

34) Despite blowing into a bag and carotid massage, a patient remains tachycardic in a narrow complex tachycardia.

35) A patient on citalopram feels unwell. The ECG notes a polymorphic tachycardia.

## Bradycardia

| | | | |
|---|---|---|---|
| a. | Atropine. | e. | Transvenous pacing. |
| b. | Glucagon. | f. | Adrenaline. |
| c. | Insulin. | g. | Observation. |
| d. | Transcutaneous pacing. | h. | No treatment. |

Match the treatment of choice for the following scenarios.

36) A patient presents with symptomatic bradycardia after an atenolol overdose.

37) A patient presents in complete heart block with dilated cardiomyopathy. They require transcutaneous pacing to maintain a heart rate above 40 bpm.

38) A patient presents in sinus bradycardia of 40 bpm. They are treated for paroxysmal AF with beta-blockers and digoxin. The patient is asymptomatic with a blood pressure of 130/70mmHg.

39) A patient has a syncopal episode, with a heart rate of 35 bpm.

40) Following percutaneous coronary intervention to the right coronary artery, a patient develops symptomatic bradycardia unresponsive to IV medication.

## Arrhythmia syndromes

a.  Brugada syndrome.                      e.  Lown-Ganong-Levine syndrome.
b.  Right ventricular dysplasia.           f.  Jervell and Lange-Nielsen syndrome.
c.  Obstructive cardiomyopathy.            g.  Romano-Ward syndrome.
d.  Wolff-Parkinson-White syndrome.        h.  Tetralogy of Fallot.

## Match the description below with the syndrome.

41) A routine medical identifies a prolonged QT interval in an otherwise healthy individual.

42) A patient presents following recurrent episodes of palpitations. There are delta waves on the ECG.

43) A 40-year-old male of Asian descent suddenly dies. The post-mortem finds a structurally normal heart.

44) A child with deaf mutism is found to have a prolonged QT interval.

45) A patient presents in the emergency department with a narrow complex tachycardia that resolves spontaneously. Repeat ECG identifies a very short PR interval with no other abnormalities on the ECG or examination.

## Short answer questions

1) A 32-year-old male attends the emergency department with central chest pain, which is worse when lying flat and relieved by sitting forwards. There is some associated shortness of breath. Pericarditis is suspected.

| | | |
|---|---|---|
| a. | Name two findings on examination. | 2 marks |
| b. | Specify one finding on this patient's ECG. | 1 mark |
| c. | Give four causes for this patient's pericarditis. | 4 marks |
| d. | Name two medications that will provide symptomatic relief. | 2 marks |
| e. | What is the single most important investigation to perform after making the clinical diagnosis of pericarditis? | 1 mark |

2) A 70-year-old male presents acutely short of breath, requiring high-flow oxygen to maintain saturations of >92%. He has had worsening exercise tolerance over several months and a recent inability to lie flat.

| | | |
|---|---|---|
| a. | Describe four typical signs on a chest X-ray for this condition. | 4 marks |
| b. | Give three underlying causes of left ventricular failure. | 3 marks |
| c. | Name one medication to treat severe pulmonary oedema in the emergency department. | 1 mark |
| d. | Name a classification system for congestive cardiac failure. | 1 mark |
| e. | Give one trigger for acute worsening of pulmonary oedema. | 1 mark |

3) A 30-year-old patient presents with night sweats and weight loss. On examination, he has track marks on his arms and a pansystolic murmur.

a.  What is the most likely organism responsible for the infection?    1 mark
b.  Which heart valve is most likely to be infected?    1 mark
c.  What is the name of the criteria used in the diagnosis of infective    1 mark
    endocarditis?
d.  Describe four risk factors for infective endocarditis.    4 marks
e.  In cases of suspected infective endocarditis, which three    3 marks
    investigations are essential?

4) A 50-year-old male presents with crushing chest pain with ST elevation in the anterior septal leads. He is treated as an ST-elevation MI.

a.  Specify four immediate management options for the patient.    4 marks
b.  Name one definitive management for this patient.    1 mark
c.  What is the most likely coronary artery that is occluded?    1 mark
d.  What is the oxygen target for this patient (assuming no other    1 mark
    respiratory disease or significant past medical history)?
e.  Name three complications of a myocardial infarction.    3 marks

5) A 54-year-old presents to the emergency department following a sudden collapse. She gives a 6-month history of worsening shortness of breath, which sometimes wakes her at night. Her brother passed away aged 46 years due to a "big heart".

a.  Specify four signs that are likely to be present on examination.    4 marks
b.  Give the next three most appropriate investigations.    3 marks
c.  What is the most likely cause of the sudden collapse?    1 mark
d.  What is the most common type of cardiac myopathy?    1 mark
e.  Name one piece of advice that should be offered on exercise.    1 mark

6) A 60-year-old patient presents to their primary care doctor with persistently elevated blood pressure of 170/100mmHg despite taking amlodipine 10mg once daily.

a. What would be the most appropriate medication to prescribe?    1 mark
b. Give four complications of untreated hypertension.    4 marks
c. Specify two pieces of lifestyle advice you would recommend.    2 marks
d. Name the risk assessment tool used for cardiovascular risk.    1 mark
e. State two blood tests that may be useful for this patient.    2 marks

7) A 65-year-old male presents to the emergency department following an episode of chest pain that came on while running for a bus. The chest pain resolved shortly after rest. He experienced similar pain previously while playing with his grandchildren. His ECG shows no acute changes and his troponin levels are not raised 6 hours following the incident. A diagnosis of stable angina is made.

a. Give three modifiable risk factors for angina pectoris.    3 marks
b. Give three non-modifiable risk factors for angina pectoris.    3 marks
c. Describe the typical nature of cardiac chest pain.    1 mark
d. State two medications used in secondary prevention.    2 marks
e. State the medication that may relieve acute angina attacks.    1 mark

8) A 70-year-old patient with suspected congestive cardiac failure undergoes a transthoracic echocardiogram. This demonstrates severe aortic stenosis.

a. Give three ways that symptomatic aortic stenosis might present.    3 marks
b. Describe the murmur associated with aortic stenosis.    2 marks
c. State three indicators of severe aortic stenosis.    3 marks
d. Which cardiac medication should be avoided in aortic stenosis?    1 mark
e. What is the definitive management of aortic stenosis?    1 mark

9) A 68-year-old male presents to the emergency department with sudden-onset dizziness and palpitations. An ECG identifies atrial fibrillation (AF) at a rate of 120 bpm.

a. What is the characteristic pulse associated with AF? 1 mark
b. Describe three characteristic features of AF with a fast ventricular response on an ECG. 3 marks
c. Name two medications to provide adequate rate control. 2 marks
d. How long should AF last before anticoagulation should be considered and what is the scoring system used to guide this decision? 2 marks
e. Name two medications used for anticoagulation in patients with AF. 2 marks

10) A 30-year-old female presents to the emergency department with palpitations. She is otherwise fit and well. Her ECG demonstrates a regular, narrow complex tachycardia.

a. Give two examples of vagal manoeuvres. 2 marks
b. Which two medications should be avoided in asthma patients? 2 marks
c. What intervention could be considered if medical therapy provides inadequate control? 1 mark
d. Name two pre-excitation syndromes that might predispose to narrow complex tachycardias. 2 marks
e. Describe three adverse features. 3 marks

11) A homeless male is found unconscious. There is a strong smell of alcohol. He is noted to be bradycardic at 30 to 40 bpm and is unarousable.

a. What is the first-line medication to treat the bradycardia? 1 mark
b. Describe three adverse features. 3 marks
c. Give four causes of non-physiological bradycardia. 4 marks
d. If medical interventions fails, what is the next appropriate step? 1 mark
e. If bradycardia persists and the patient remains symptomatic, what would be the definitive management? 1 mark

12) A 12-year-old boy presents to the emergency department with chest pain and fever. He recently arrived from Somalia. Two weeks ago he had had a sore throat. His mother is unsure about previous vaccinations. The ECG is consistent with myocarditis.

| | | |
|---|---|---|
| a. | Which bacteria are associated with rheumatic fever? | 1 mark |
| b. | Name the diagnostic criteria used to diagnosis rheumatic fever. | 1 mark |
| c. | Describe three cardiac sequelae of rheumatic fever. | 3 marks |
| d. | Give two medications that are useful in managing this patient. | 2 marks |
| e. | Name three non-cardiac features of rheumatic fever. | 3 marks |

13) A patient collapses shortly after undergoing percutaneous coronary intervention. The patient is not breathing and there is no palpable central pulse.

| | | |
|---|---|---|
| a. | Give two causes of reversible cardiac causes of cardiac arrest. | 2 marks |
| b. | Name two shockable rhythms. | 2 marks |
| c. | Name two non-shockable rhythms. | 2 marks |
| d. | What is the ratio of chest compressions to ventilations? | 1 mark |
| e. | Name the two medications used during cardiac pulmonary resuscitation, if there are no reversible causes, and at what point they are given. | 3 marks |

# Chapter 2

# Respiratory
## QUESTIONS

## Single best answer questions

1) A 60-year-old patient presents to the emergency department with a cough, which is productive of green sputum, and fevers. Chest radiograph identifies an area of consolidation in the right lower zone. The patient is normally fit and well, without any allergies. Observations are stable. Blood tests demonstrate an elevated CRP and neutrophilia only. What is the choice of antibiotics at discharge from the department?

a. Amoxicillin.
b. Co-amoxiclav.
c. Clarithromycin.
d. Doxycycline.

2) A 70-year-old male presents with a productive cough, confusion and fevers. His blood pressure is 90/65mmHg, respiratory rate 20, SpO$_2$ 93% on air, heart rate 100 beats per minute, temperature 39°C. Blood results are as follows: Hb 130g/L, WCC 16 x 10$^9$/L, platelets 300 x 10$^9$/L, Na$^+$ 137mmol/L, K$^+$ 5.3mmol/L, urea 9mmol/L, creatinine 180μmol/L. He is normally independent and well. What is his CURB-65 score?

a. 1.
b. 2.
c. 3.
d. 4.

3) A 65-year-old male with a history of alcohol excess presents with a lower respiratory tract infection. Which causative organism is classically associated with alcohol use?

a. *Klebsiella pneumoniae.*
b. *Legionella pneumophila.*
c. *Moraxella catarrhalis.*
d. *Streptococcus pneumoniae.*

4) A patient presents to their primary care doctor with shortness of breath, wheeze and cough at night despite taking the regular maximum dose of inhaled beclomethasone. They are frequently using their salbutamol inhaler. What is the next step in management?

a. Oral steroids.
b. Regular inhaled long-acting beta-agonist.
c. Regular inhaled short-acting beta-agonist.
d. Regular inhaled short-acting anti-muscarinic.

5) A patient presents with a productive cough. The sputum is rusty-coloured. What is the most likely causative organism?

a. *Klebsiella pneumomiae.*
b. *Legionella pneumophila.*
c. *Moraxella catarrhalis.*
d. *Streptococcus pneumoniae.*

6) A 21-year-old male, previously fit and well, presents with pleuritic chest pain and shortness of breath. There is no history of trauma. Chest radiograph shows a 3cm pneumothorax measured at the height of the mediastinum. What is the next most appropriate step?

a. Aspiration.
b. High-flow oxygen.
c. Insert a chest drain.
d. Observation for 24 hours.

7) A 30-year-old female presents with shortness of breath to the emergency department. She is concerned that she might have a pulmonary embolism. Which tool is most useful to exclude a pulmonary embolism?

a. PERC criteria.
b. Wells score for DVT.
c. Wells score for PE.
d. Z-score.

8) A patient known to have asthma presents with severe shortness of breath. Which of the following are suggestive of a life-threatening asthma attack?

a. Heart rate 113 bpm.
b. Peak expiratory flow rate 35% of best.
c. An inability to form a complete sentence in one breath.
d. Normal $PaCO_2$.

9) A 70-year-old patient presents with acute shortness of breath on a background of COPD. There are bilateral wheezes on auscultation and there are no acute changes on chest radiograph. What are the most appropriate medications to prescribe?

a. Salbutamol INH, ipratropium INH, prednisolone, doxycycline.
b. Salbutamol NEB, ipratropium NEB, prednisolone, amoxicillin.
c. Salbutamol NEB, ipratropium NEB, hydrocortisone, amoxicillin.
d. Salbutamol NEB, ipratropium NEB, prednisolone, doxycycline.

10) A patient with COPD develops a pneumothorax. On chest radiograph, the pneumothorax is measured as 3cm from the mediastinum. What is the most appropriate management?

a. Aspiration.
b. Chest drain.
c. High-flow oxygen.
d. Lung reduction.

11) A patient presents to the emergency department with shortness of breath and weight loss. Their past medical history includes intravenous drug use and asthma as a

child. The chest radiograph is clear. At rest $SpO_2$ is >94% but on exertion there is marked oxygen desaturation. What is the most likely diagnosis?

a. Chronic untreated asthma.
b. *Mycobacterium spp.* pneumonia.
c. Pneumoconiosis.
d. *Pneumocystis jirovecii.*

12) Despite salbutamol and ipratropium nebulisers, IV hydrocortisone and empirical antibiotics, a patient with a severe exacerbation of COPD continues to deteriorate. The latest ABG results are: $PaO_2$ 5kPa, $PaCO_2$ 10kPa, pH 7.3, lactate 2mmol/L. What is the next step in management?

a. Further salbutamol nebuliser.
b. High-flow oxygen.
c. Intubation.
d. Non-invasive ventilation.

13) A 50-year-old male presents with haemoptysis and a severe acute kidney injury is found on blood tests. There is a saddle nose deformity and bilateral crepitations on examination. What is the most likely diagnosis?

a. Alport syndrome.
b. Goodpasture's syndrome.
c. Granulomatosis with polyangiitis.
d. *Mycobacterium tuberculosis.*

14) A patient with lung sarcoidosis is reviewed in clinic. A routine chest radiograph is performed which shows bilaterally hilar lymphadenopathy and bilateral infiltrates. Specify the stage of pulmonary sarcoidosis.

a.   Stage 1.
b.   Stage 2.
c.   Stage 3.
d.   Stage 4.

15) A 49-year-old female presenting with shortness of breath is found to have a right-sided pleural effusion. Aspiration of the fluid finds this to be transudative. Blood results are within the normal range. The patient is currently under investigation for an ovarian mass that appears benign in origin without any other previous health problems. What is the most likely underlying cause for the pleural effusion?

a.   Congestive cardiac failure.
b.   Hypothyroidism.
c.   Malignancy.
d.   Meigs' syndrome.

16) A 65-year-old male presents with a history of fatigue, waking during the night, snoring and headaches in the morning. These symptoms have been gradually worsening over several years. Examination is unremarkable with the exception of a large habitus. What is the most likely underlying diagnosis?

a.   Asthma.
b.   Congestive cardiac failure.
c.   Obstructive sleep apnoea.
d.   Pulmonary fibrosis.

17) A 65-year-old patient presents with a bothersome cough for several weeks. The sputum varies in colour. The past medical history is unremarkable except for recurrent chest infections as a child. On examination, the JVP is at 6cm, the chest is resonant to percussion throughout and there are bilateral crepitations (right side greater than left). There is pitting oedema to the knees bilaterally. What is the most likely diagnosis?

a.   Bronchiectasis.
b.   Bronchiectasis with pulmonary hypertension.
c.   Congestive cardiac disease.
d.   Lung fibrosis.

18) Which of the following medications used in smoking cessation is contraindicated in patients with epilepsy?

a.   Bupropion.
b.   Nicotine gum.
c.   Nicotine patches.
d.   Varenicline.

19) A 1-year-old child is seen in the respiratory clinic for recurrent chest infections with purulent sputum. The child has a past medical history of meconium ileus and evidence of a failure to thrive. What is the underlying diagnosis?

a.   Bronchiolitis.
b.   Bronchiectasis.
c.   Cystic fibrosis.
d.   Asthma.

20) A 23-year-old asthmatic presents to his primary care doctor for an asthma review. His peak flow is mildly reduced compared with his previous review last year and he is using his salbutamol inhaler more frequently. He has no other medication. What would be the next appropriate treatment for this patient?

a. Salbutamol and beclomethasone inhalers.
b. Salbutamol and salmeterol inhalers.
c. Beclomethasone inhaler only.
d. Stop salbutamol.

21) A 24-year-old male arrives in the emergency department with shortness of breath. A chest X-ray is performed. What does this image show?

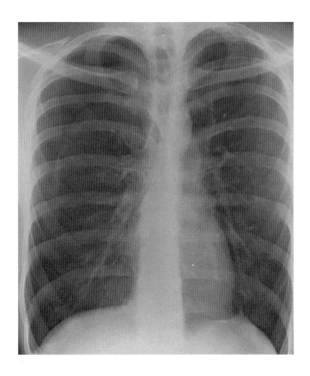

a.  Left lower lobe collapse.
b.  Normal chest X-ray.
c.  Right pneumothorax.
d.  Right tension pneumothorax.

22) A 24-year-old female is reviewed by his primary care doctor with a 6-week history of progressive shortness of breath. A chest X-ray is taken to investigate symptoms. What does this image show?

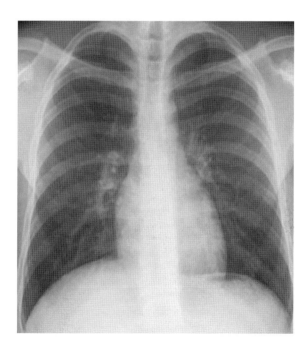

a.  Right middle lung lesion.
b.  Right pneumothorax.
c.  Normal chest X-ray.
d.  Right pleural effusion.

23) A 62-year-old male presents to his his primary care doctor with a 6-week history of haemoptysis and shortness of breath. A chest X-ray is performed which shows a lesion suspicious of malignancy. In which lobe is this located?

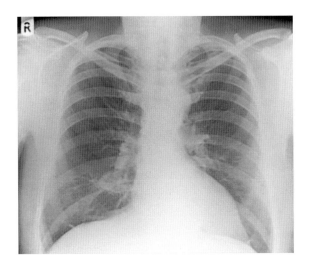

a.   Right upper lobe.
b.   Right middle lobe.
c.   Right lower lobe.
d.   Left upper lobe.

# Extended matching questions

## Examination findings

a.    Lower respiratory infection.      e.    Pleural effusion.

b.    Upper respiratory infection.      f.    Emphysema.

c.    Collapsed lobe.                    g.    Asthma.

d.    Pneumothorax.                      h.    Bronchiectasis.

Select the most likely diagnosis for the examination findings below.

1)    Clubbing, symmetrical chest expansion, bilateral fine crepitation.

2)    Reduced chest expansion on the right, trachea deviated to the right, dull to percussion on the right, reduced air entry on the right, no added sounds.

3)    Reduced chest expansion on the right, trachea deviated to the left, stony dull to percussion on the right, reduced air entry on the right, no added sounds.

4)    Hyper-expanded chest, tar staining on fingers, hyper-resonant to percussion, poor entry throughout lung fields, bilateral wheeze.

5)    Reduced chest expansion on the right, trachea deviated to the left, hyper-resonant to percussion at the right apex, decreased air sounds on the right.

## History of respiratory illness in the young

a.  Lower respiratory infection.   e.  Pleural effusion.
b.  Upper respiratory infection.   f.  Cystic fibrosis.
c.  Collapsed lobe.                g.  Asthma.
d.  Pneumothorax.                  h.  Bronchiectasis.

Match the description of the patient with the most likely diagnosis.

6)  A 25-year-old patient presents with a cough at night and worsening exercise tolerance since moving to a new address.

7)  A 20-year-old current smoker presents with sudden-onset sharp chest pain, which is worse on inspiration, and an associated shortness of breath.

8)  A 6-year-old with a history of recurrent chest infections presents with a productive cough. He is of Pakistani descent and his parents are first cousins. He has marked clubbing.

9)  A 25-year-old presents with headaches, cough and rhinorrhoea. There is no history of fevers.

10) A 30-year-old female with a history of rheumatoid arthritis presents with a productive cough and fevers.

## History of respiratory illness in the elderly

| | | | |
|---|---|---|---|
| a. | Lower respiratory infection. | e. | Lung carcinoma. |
| b. | Upper respiratory infection. | f. | COPD. |
| c. | Pulmonary oedema. | g. | Tuberculosis. |
| d. | Idiopathic fibrosis. | h. | Bronchiectasis. |

Match the description of the patient with the most likely diagnosis.

11) A 75-year-old female originally from Romania presents with weight loss and a cough having started systemic treatment for bullous pemphigoid.

12) A 65-year-old presents with increasing shortness of breath over several weeks which is not worse on lying flat. He has noticed odd nail changes.

13) An 80-year-old presents with a productive cough and an increasing shortness of breath over several months. She has a history of tuberculosis as a child and recurrent chest infections.

14) A 70-year-old male presents with severe constipation, weight loss and a dry cough gradually developing over 4 weeks. He was previously very active.

15) An 85-year-old patient has noticed worsening breathlessness over several weeks. This is worse at night and she has found that she needs more pillows to sleep comfortably at night. She has also generally felt more tired.

## Pneumonia: causative organisms

a.  *Streptococcus pneumoniae.*  e.  *Legionella spp.*

b.  *Staphylococcus aureus.*  f.  *Chlamydia pneumoniae.*

c.  *Klebsiella spp.*  g.  *Chlamydia psittaci.*

d.  *Mycoplasma spp.*  h.  *Pneumocystis jirovecii.*

## Match the presentation to the most likely causative organism.

16) A 65-year-old male is making a good recovery from influenza when he suddenly develops severe shortness of breath and a productive cough.

17) A patient presents with a dry cough and rash following a period of flu-like symptoms. The rash looks like a series of red bull's eye targets.

18) A patient returns from a Mediterranean holiday and develops loose stools and a dry cough.

19) A patient develops a dry cough shortly after purchasing a parrot.

20) A 75-year-old patient develops a productive cough and fever.

## Pneumonia: complications

a.  Atrial fibrillation.               e.  Severe sepsis.
b.  Empyema.                          f.  Septic shock.
c.  Parapneumonic effusion.          g.  ARDS.
d.  Sepsis.                           h.  Lung abscess.

Match the description of the patient with the most likely complication.

21) A patient is making a good recovery from a lower respiratory chest infection caused by *Staphylococcus aureus* when they develop a recurrent fever. There is new stony dullness to percussion over the right lung.

22) A patient presents with a severe lower respiratory tract infection. On percussion, there is stony dull percussion adjacent to coarse crepitations. As the chest infection resolves, the area of stony dullness improves.

23) An intravenous drug user presents with shortness of breath and a cough. The sputum is foul and purulent with occasional streaks of blood.

24) A patient presents with confusion, a productive cough and shortness of breath. Despite aggressive IV fluids, blood pressure remains low.

25) A patient presents with confusion, a productive cough and shortness of breath. There is anuria, tachycardia and hypotension, responding to fluids.

## Hypersensitivity pneumonitis

| | | | |
|---|---|---|---|
| a. | *Aspergillus clavatus.* | e. | *Penicillium casei.* |
| b. | Avian antigens. | f. | *Pseudomonas aeruginosa.* |
| c. | *Botrytis.* | g. | *Streptococcus pneumoniae.* |
| d. | *Micropolyspora faeni.* | h. | *Thermophilic actinomycetes.* |

Match the hypersensitivity pneumonitis with the causative factor.

26) Bird fancier's lung.

27) Malt worker's lung.

28) Farmer's lung.

29) Mushroom worker's disease.

30) Wine maker's lung.

## Lung malignancy: classification

a. Adenocarcinoma.

b. Carcinoid tumour.

c. Hamartoma.

d. Large-cell carcinoma.

e. Mesothelioma.

f. Metastasis.

g. Small cell carcinoma.

h. Squamous cell carcinoma.

Match the presentation with the most likely underlying malignancy.

31) A peripheral lung lesion is an incidental finding on a chest radiograph in an otherwise well 65-year-old female, who is a life-long non-smoker.

32) A 50-year-old male, heavy life-long smoker, presents with severe constipation and has a centrally positioned lung lesion on X-ray.

33) A 70-year-old male presents with severe bone pain, a dry cough and weight loss. He has a raised blood pressure with purple abdominal striae.

34) A 55-year-old boiler engineer presents with shortness of breath and he is found to have a unilateral pleural effusion. He is a life-long non-smoker and has no other significant past medical history.

35) A chest X-ray is performed on a patient who presents with shortness of breath. There are multiple circular lesions bilaterally across lung fields.

## Lung malignancy: complications

a. Bony metastasis.
b. Paraneoplastic syndrome.
c. Venous thromboembolism.
d. SVC obstruction.
e. Horner's syndrome.
f. Phrenic nerve palsy.
g. Laryngeal nerve palsy.
h. Ataxia.

Match the complication of lung malignancy with the presentation.

36) A patient presents with distended neck veins and shortness of breath.

37) A patient presents with chest pain, shortness of breath and palpitations.

38) A patient presents with severe pain in his chest, back and left hip. He is currently awaiting a 2-week referral for suspected lung malignancy.

39) A frail elderly patient has the incidental finding of a raised hemi-diaphragm on chest radiograph and a restrictive pattern of breathing on spirometry but denies any symptoms at present.

40) A patient presents with shoulder pain and is noted to have miosis and ptosis.

## Interstitial lung disease

| | | | |
|---|---|---|---|
| a. | Amiodarone. | e. | Scleroderma. |
| b. | Asbestosis. | f. | Seronegative arthropathy. |
| c. | Bleomycin. | g. | Silica. |
| d. | Coal. | h. | Tuberculosis. |

Match the description of the patient with the most likely causative agent.

41) A patient is undergoing chemotherapy when they develop a gradual onset of shortness of breath.

42) A 20-year-old patient presents with progressive shortness of breath. There are basal fine inspiratory crepitations on examination.

43) A 25-year-old patient presents with mild shortness of breath. There are apical crepitations on examination.

44) A 55-year-old ex-miner presents with severe shortness of breath with massive mid and upper zone fibrosis on a high-resolution CT.

45) A 45-year-old male presents with worsening shortness of breath. He has a history of dilated cardiac myopathy and associated ventricular tachycardia. Despite diuretic therapy, there are persistent lower zone crepitations.

## Short answer questions

1) A 35-year-old Afro-Caribbean presents with shortness of breath and a dry cough. She gives a 3-week history of painful joints. A chest X-ray shows bilateral hilar lymphadenopathy and pulmonary infiltrates. Sarcoidosis is suspected.

a. Give two other causes of bilateral hilar lymphadenopathy.    2 marks
b. Give two skin manifestations of sarcoidosis.    2 marks
c. What is the characteristic finding on histology for sarcoidosis?    1 mark
d. What finding on lung function tests is seen in sarcoidosis?    1 mark
e. Specify the results of four blood tests used to diagnose sarcoidosis.    4 marks

2) A 30-year-old homeless male presents with weight loss, haemoptysis and shortness of breath developing over several weeks. There is unilateral cervical lymphadenopathy. Tuberculosis is suspected.

a. The lymph node is biopsied and there are granulomas on histology.    3 marks
   Other than sarcoid and TB, list three granulomatous diseases.
b. Name the four antibiotics prescribed in tuberculosis.    4 marks
c. Which stain is used to help identify *Mycobacterium spp.*?    1 mark
d. Describe another technique used in diagnosing tuberculosis.    1 mark
e. What media is used for culturing *Mycobacterium spp.*?    1 mark

3) A 25-year-old female presents acutely short of breath with pleuritic chest pain. Her heart rate is 125 bpm and her blood pressure is 80/50mmHg. It is noted that she has a painful swollen left calf muscle. A PE is suspected.

a. What is the gold standard investigation for diagnosis of a PE?    1 mark
b. What is the treatment of choice for this patient?    1 mark
c. What is the complication of recurrent or untreated PE?    1 mark
d. Name four risk factors for pulmonary embolism.    4 marks
e. Describe three typical patterns on ECGs for PE.    3 marks

4) A 65-year-old male with COPD presents with shortness of breath. There is a bilateral wheeze on auscultation and there is no focal consolidation on chest radiograph. The patient is diagnosed with an acute exacerbation of COPD.

a. What three medications should be given acutely to this patient?    3 marks
b. What other measures can be taken should initial therapy fail to resolve the acute exacerbation of COPD?    3 marks
c. What are the two classical pictures of COPD?    2 marks
d. Other than a chest radiograph, what is the most important investigation in the management of a patient with COPD?    1 mark
e. What surgical interventions can be used to manage COPD?    1 mark

5) An 18-year-old male presents with a life-threatening asthma attack. He normally uses a preventer and reliever inhaler only. He has no other medical history.

| | | |
|---|---|---|
| a. | State four features suggestive of a life-threatening asthma attack. | 4 marks |
| b. | Name three IV drugs used to treat acute asthma exacerbations. | 3 marks |
| c. | Name one complication of ventilation requiring high pressures. | 1 mark |
| d. | What oxygen delivery system should be used first line? | 1 mark |
| e. | The patient makes a good recovery and he is able to be discharged. What one medication must the patient be discharged with? | 1 mark |

6) A 20-year-old patient with cystic fibrosis presents with worsening shortness of breath and a cough. He is pyrexial on admission and appears unwell.

| | | |
|---|---|---|
| a. | Describe two signs found in patients with cystic fibrosis. | 2 marks |
| b. | Name three organisms associated with cystic fibrosis. | 2 marks |
| c. | Name two methods used in the diagnosis of cystic fibrosis. | 2 marks |
| d. | Describe three complications outside the respiratory system. | 3 marks |
| e. | Name the inheritance pattern of cystic fibrosis. | 1 mark |

7) A 75-year-old male is admitted with shortness of breath, a productive cough and confusion. The patient has no allergies. His chest radiograph shows focal consolidation in the right base. Chest sepsis is diagnosed.

| | | |
|---|---|---|
| a. | As part of Sepsis Six, what three things must be taken or measured? | 3 marks |
| b. | As part of Sepsis Six, what three things must be given? | 3 marks |
| c. | *Streptococcus pneumoniae* is suspected. What is the typical sputum? | 1 mark |
| d. | What is the most appropriate first-line medication? | 1 mark |
| e. | Describe two findings on examination. | 2 marks |

8) A young male is found unresponsive outside a railway station. Cyanosis is evident despite high-flow oxygen with a respiratory rate of 30 breaths per minute. He is hot to touch and track marks are present on his arms and legs with associated abscesses. On auscultation there are fine crepitations. The team suspects acute respiratory distress syndrome (ARDS).

a. Where should this patient be managed?     1 mark
b. Name five causes of ARDS.     5 marks
c. What is the most likely finding on chest radiograph?     1 mark
d. Name two risks associated with artificial ventilation.     2 marks
e. What is the prognosis in ARDS?     1 mark

9) A 70-year-old male presents with shortness of breath. He is known to have cryptogenic lung fibrosis. An ABG identifies Type 2 respiratory failure.

a. Describe three signs or symptoms caused by hypercapnia.     3 marks
b. Define Type 2 respiratory failure.     2 marks
c. What should the oxygen target be?     1 mark
d. Describe two oxygen delivery methods for achieving this target.     2 marks
e. Once stable, what two signs are likely to be found in this patient?     2 marks

10) A 55-year-old business male is referred for sleep studies and respiratory outpatients by his primary care doctor, who suspects obstructive sleep apnoea.

a. Describe three risk factors for obstructive sleep apnoea.     3 marks
b. Describe three clinical features for this condition.     3 marks
c. Describe two lifestyle advice measures that should be offered.     2 marks
d. Name one other intervention that might be offered.     1 mark
e. Specify one surgical intervention used in managing this condition.     1 mark

11) A 45-year-old male with chronic asthma, requiring multiple courses of oral steroids, presents with a persistent cough and wheeze despite optimising medical management. He has chronic sinusitis. Further investigations are positive for *Aspergillus spp.* serology.

a. Name four respiratory diseases associated with *Aspergillus*. 4 marks
b. Other than steroids, what can be used to manage the *Aspergillus* colonisation of the respiratory system? 1 mark
c. What might the chest X-ray or CT scans identify? 1 mark
d. Describe three complications of long-term steroid use. 3 marks
e. What other blood tests might support the diagnosis? 1 mark

12) A 77-year-old female presents with worsening shortness of breath. Her chest radiograph has findings consistent with a right-sided unilateral pleural effusion. She is referred to the respiratory medicine department for further investigation.

a. Give two signs consistent with a pleural effusion. 2 marks
b. Describe the appearance of a pleural effusion on chest X-ray. 1 mark
c. Name the criteria used in distinguishing exudates from transudates. 1 mark
d. Other than biochemistry, give two other tests that should be performed on an aspirate sample. 2 marks
e. The pleural effusion is confirmed as an exudate. Name four differential diagnoses for the cause of the exudate. 4 marks

13) An 82-year-old female presents with a difficulty in breathing. Her neck veins are congested and she appears plethoric. She has a background of ischaemic heart disease and rheumatoid arthritis, and is an ex-smoker. There is a suspicion of superior vena cava obstruction.

a.  Describe Pemberton's sign.                                                    1 mark
b.  What is the typical distribution of peripheral oedema?                         1 mark
c.  List four possible causes of superior vena cava obstruction.                   4 marks
d.  What is the most likely cause of superior vena cava obstruction in this        1 mark
    patient?
e.  State three approaches for alleviating the obstruction.                        3 marks

# Chapter 3

# Gastroenterology
## QUESTIONS

## Single best answer questions

1) A 25-year-old female who has recently emigrated to the UK from Zimbabwe presents to her primary care doctor with dry eyes and night blindness. On examination, collections of keratin in the conjunctiva are noted. Her doctor believes she has a vitamin deficiency. Which vitamin deficiency would cause the patient's symptoms?

a. Vitamin A.
b. Vitamin $B_3$.
c. Folate.
d. Vitamin E.

2) A 68-year-old male presents to his primary care doctor with a 6-week history of fatigue, pallor and shortness of breath. A full blood count shows a mild anaemia with haematinics showing a normal serum iron but low vitamin $B_{12}$. He is referred to a gastroenterologist who suspects the patient has pernicious anaemia. What test could be performed to confirm the diagnosis?

a. Barium meal.
b. Non-invasive liver screen.
c. Schilling test.
d. Rapid urease test.

3) A 25-year-old male with a history of bulimia attends the emergency department with three episodes of haematemesis. He does not drink alcohol and has had multiple episodes of vomiting for the past 24 hours. He vomits once whilst you are examining him which is blood-stained. On examination, he is tachycardic, clammy and has a blood pressure of 100/80mmHg. He undergoes fluid resuscitation in the emergency department and an endoscopy is performed which reveals the cause of his haematemesis. What is the most likely finding in this patient?

a. Oesophageal varices.
b. Mallory-Weiss syndrome.
c. Haemorrhagic gastritis.
d. Peptic ulcer disease.

4) A 42-year-old female presents to her primary care doctor with recurrent abdominal pain for the past 6 months. She states that the pain is present most days and pain is improved following defecation. She feels bloated and bowel movements are increased compared with 12 months ago. She has been reviewed by her doctor several times and investigations are unremarkable. She has a history of anxiety. What is the most likely diagnosis?

a. Crohn's disease.
b. Ulcerative colitis.
c. Irritable bowel syndrome.
d. Ovarian cancer.

5) A 56-year-old male is referred from his primary care doctor with a 2-month history of dysphagia; symptoms occur with both solids and liquids. He has also noted chest pain, weight loss and a cough. Chest X-ray reveals a fluid level in the oesophagus and loss of the gastric bubble. A barium swallow demonstrates oesophageal dilatation and a bird's beak appearance in the distal oesophagus. What is the most likely diagnosis?

a. Achalasia.
b. Oesophageal spasm.
c. Hiatus hernia.
d. Gastro-oesophageal reflux disease.

6)  A 45-year-old alcoholic male is brought into the emergency department by an ambulance crew after they found him wandering around the streets in a confused state. He is unable to give a history. On examination, you note ophthalmoplegia and ataxia of his upper and lower limbs. You suspect that this is a complication of alcohol withdrawal. What is the most likely diagnosis?

a.  Delirium tremens.
b.  Korsakoff psychosis.
c.  Hypoglycaemia.
d.  Wernicke's encephalopathy.

7)  A 28-year-old male with autoimmune hepatitis presents to the emergency department with a 12-hour history of nausea, anorexia and fatigue. His partner is concerned he is confused and does not recognise his surroundings. On examination, he is jaundiced and displays asterixis. What is the most likely diagnosis?

a.  Hepatic encephalopathy.
b.  Alcohol withdrawal.
c.  Liver failure.
d.  Gallstones.

8)  A 25-year-old final year medical student is attending occupational health as part of his health clearance for the Foundation Training Programme. His results confirm that he is immune to Hepatitis B due to vaccination. Which of the following will be positive to confirm immunity due to vaccination?

a.    Hepatitis B surface antigen (HBsAg).
b.    Hepatitis B surface antibody (anti-HBs).
c.    Hepatitis B core antibody (anti-HBc).
d.    Hepatitis B e antigen (HBeAg).

9)    A 52-year-old male is admitted to the gastroenterology ward with jaundice. He has had several previous admissions and the gastroenterologist requests a liver biopsy; this shows the presence of inclusion bodies in the cytoplasm of liver cells. The gastroenterologist informs the medical students that this is Mallory's hyaline. What is the most likely diagnosis?

a.    Ischaemic disease.
b.    Hepatitis infection.
c.    Alcoholic liver disease.
d.    Haemochromatosis.

10)   An 82-year-old female is admitted to the care of the elderly ward following a fall at home. She undergoes a Malnutrition Universal Screening Tool (MUST) assessment which shows she has not eaten in 10 days and prior to this her diet consisted of custard and biscuits. She is reviewed by a dietician who advises that artificial nutrition is required and daily bloods to be taken. What complication of artificial nutrition are they concerned about?

a.    Refeeding syndrome.
b.    Acute pancreatitis.
c.    Liver failure.
d.    Hyperglycaemia.

11) A 32-year-old male presents to his primary care doctor with shortness of breath, tiredness and fatigue. He was previously fit and well prior to this episode and has no past medical history. On examination, he is pale and noted to have glossitis, angular cheilitis and koilonychia. Blood tests reveal a hypochromic microcytic anaemia with a low ferritin. What is the underlying diagnosis?

a.  Iron deficiency anaemia.
b.  Folate deficiency anaemia.
c.  $B_{12}$ deficiency anaemia.
d.  Anaemia of chronic disease.

12) Thumb printing would be seen on the plain abdominal X-ray in all of the following cases other than which condition?

a.  Ischaemic colitis.
b.  Diverticular disease.
c.  Ulcerative colitis.
d.  Crohn's disease.

13) A 42-year-old male presents to her primary care doctor with a 2-month history of dyspepsia and intermittent epigastric pain that occurs after food. He has noticed recently that he has a dry cough in the morning. He denies any weight loss, dysphagia or vomiting. He is otherwise fit and well. What is the underylying diagnosis?

a.  Oesophageal web.
b.  Oesophageal carcinoma.
c.  Gastro-oesophageal reflux disease.
d.  Barrett's oesophagus.

14) A 32-year-old female is referred to a gastroenterologist following a 2-month history of diarrhoea, steatorrhoea and abdominal pain. Blood tests reveal an iron deficiency anaemia. The gastroenterologist requests tissue transglutaminase antibodies which are positive. Endoscopic duodenal biopsies show villous atrophy and crypt hyperplasia. What is the underlying diagnosis?

a.   Lactose intolerance.
b.   Coeliac disease.
c.   Gastroenteritis.
d.   Carcinoid tumour.

15) A 43-year-old male is admitted to the emergency department with a 5-day history of abdominal pain and profuse diarrhoea. He underwent a circumcision for phimosis complicated by a wound infection 2 weeks ago for which he was given two different courses of antibiotics. On examination, he is dehydrated and has a mild pyrexia. Stool culture is positive for a Gram-positive rod. What is the most likely diagnosis?

a.   *Staphylococcus aureus.*
b.   *Shigella spp.*
c.   *Streptococcus pyogenes.*
d.   *Clostridium difficile.*

16) A 32-year-old male is admitted to the gastroenterology ward with severe bloody diarrhoea and abdominal pain. He is having five bowel motions per day. On examination, he has a fever of 38.2°C and is tachycardic. He is known to have ulcerative colitis. What is the first-line therapy?

a. IV hydrocortisone.
b. IV antibiotics.
c. Methotrexate.
d. Infliximab.

17) A 56-year-old female underwent a laparoscopic cholecystectomy 6 weeks ago and attends her primary care doctor due to multiple episodes of diarrhoea for the past 4 weeks. She denies any unusual foods, foreign travel or weight loss. On examination, she appears well with an unremarkable examination. Her doctor thinks the patient has post-cholecystectomy syndrome and the diarrhoea is a result of bile acid malabsorption and prescribes a bile acid sequestrant. What is the most likely medication prescribed for this patient?

a. Ursodeoxycholic acid.
b. Cholestyramine.
c. Paracetamol.
d. Chlorphenamine.

18) A 43-year-old alcoholic male is admitted to the emergency department following a fall in which he sustains a fracture to his left arm. He is admitted to the ward for further management. He is prescribed a reducing dose of chlordiazepoxide to manage alcohol withdrawal. What

other medication should be prescribed to prevent Wernicke's encephalopathy?

a. Disulfiram.
b. Acamprosate.
c. Naltrexone.
d. Pabrinex®.

19) A 64-year-old male is admitted following a 2-day history of painless jaundice. He has had epigastric pain for several weeks radiating to the back which is worst on lying down. He has lost 2 stone in weight over the past 6 weeks. He has never had any of these symptoms prior to this episode. On examination, he is jaundiced with a palpable gallbladder. What is the underlying diagnosis?

a. Pancreatic carcinoma.
b. Acute pancreatitis.
c. Chronic pancreatitis.
d. Cholangiocarcinoma.

20) A 1-month-old baby is admitted to the emergency department with non-bilious projectile vomiting following feeding. On examination, the patient is dehydrated and an olive mass is felt in the epigastrium. The doctor suspects pyloric stenosis. What metabolic abnormality is associated with this condition?

a. Hypochloraemic hypokalaemic metabolic alkalosis.
b. Hypochloraemic hypokalaemic metabolic acidosis.
c. Hyperchloraemic hypokalaemic metabolic alkalosis.
d. Hypochloraemic hyperkalaemic metabolic acidosis.

21) A 42-year-old male is admitted to the emergency department with abdominal pain, distention and vomiting. He has seen his primary care doctor for joint pain and headaches. On examination, he is pyrexial and has lymphadenopathy. He undergoes endoscopy showing pale yellow shaggy mucosa with erythematous eroded patches. A biopsy shows PAS-positive macrophages in the lamina propria containing Gram-positive bacilli. What is the diagnosis?

a.   Tropical sprue.
b.   Coeliac disease.
c.   Whipple's disease.
d.   Lactose intolerance.

22) A 72-year-old male with known AF is admitted with a 12-hour history of severe abdominal pain. The pain is located on the left iliac fossa and he has noted several episodes of bloody diarrhoea. On examination, he has generalised abdominal tenderness and bloods reveal a raised WCC and raised lactate. Abdominal X-ray shows thumb printing of the descending colon. What is the most likely diagnosis?

a.   Diverticulitis.
b.   Ischaemic colitis.
c.   Ulcerative colitis.
d.   Crohn's disease.

23) A 26-year-old male attends his primary care doctor with epigastric pain which is relieved by food. He had had mild nausea and vomiting but is otherwise well. What is the underlying diagnosis?

a. Barrett's oesophagus.
b. Gastro-oesophageal reflux disease.
c. Gastric ulcer.
d. Duodenal ulcer.

# Extended matching questions

## Upper gastrointestinal bleeding

a.  Oesophageal varices.          e.  Reflux oesophagitis.
b.  Mallory-Weiss syndrome.       f.  NSAIDs.
c.  Peptic ulcer.                  g.  Steroids.
d.  Aorto-enteric fistula.         h.  Gastric cancer.

Match the description of the patient with the most likely cause of their bleeding.

1)  A 52-year-old homeless gentleman with haematemesis. On examination he is jaundiced with hepatomegaly and gross ascites.

2)  A 72-year-old presents with a 24-hour history of haematemesis and malaena. He underwent an AAA repair 2 months ago. He is tachycardic and hypotensive.

3)  A 32-year-old presents with coffee ground vomiting. He has had dull epigastric pain for 6 weeks, which is worse on eating. He does not take any medication.

4)  A 19-year-old student presents to the emergency department with a 24-hour history of vomiting bright red blood. He has been vomiting for 12 hours.

5)  An 82-year-old presents with a 3-month history of epigastric pain, weight loss and early satiety. He had a previous *H. pylori* infection. On examination, he has epigastric pain and an enlarged lymph node in the left supraclavicular fossa.

## Oesophageal pathology

a.   Gastro-oesophageal reflux disease.  e.   Oesophageal carcinoma.

b.   Barrett's oesophagus.              f.   Systemic scleroderma.

c.   Hiatus hernia.                     g.   Diffuse oesophageal spasm.

d.   Achalasia.                         h.   Foreign body.

Match the description of the patient with the most likely diagnosis.

6)   A 72-year-old male presents with a 5-month history of progressive dysphagia to solids and recently to liquids. He is an ex-smoker who smoked 30 cigarettes a day for 55 years. He has lost 2 stone over the past 3 months.

7)   A 42-year-old complains of dysphagia occurring with solids and liquids. He notes chest pain and a cough. A barium swallow shows a bird's beak appearance.

8)   A 55-year-old female visits her primary care doctor with progressive dysphagia and a cough, alongside swollen and stiff fingers. On examination, she has localised finger thickening, calcinosis and telangiectasia. She is known to have Raynaud's syndrome.

9)   A 40-year-old male attends his primary care doctor with 12 months of intermittent dysphagia. He has a burning sensation and discomfort in his chest following eating relieved by belching. Chest X-ray shows a gas bubble and fluid level behind the heart.

10)  A 56-year-old attends clinic with retrosternal chest pain and intermittent dysphagia to solids and liquids. A barium swallow shows a corkscrew appearance.

## Jaundice

| | | | |
|---|---|---|---|
| a. | Crigler-Najjar syndrome. | e. | Hepatitis C. |
| b. | Gilbert's syndrome. | f. | Sickle cell crisis. |
| c. | Primary sclerosing cholangitis. | g. | Ascending cholangitis. |
| d. | Hepatitis A. | h. | Pancreatic carcinoma. |

Match the description with the most likely cause of the patient's jaundice.

11) A 32-year-old female presents to the emergency department with right upper quadrant pain and jaundice for 24 hours. On examination, she is pyrexial at 38.7°C, tachycardic and jaundiced.

12) A 60-year-old male presents with a 4-month history of painless jaundice, weight loss and epigastric pain. He has pale stools and dark urine. On examination, the gallbladder is palpable but non-tender.

13) A 32-year-old male is referred from his primary care doctor with a 3-week history of right upper quadrant pain, fatigue, weight loss and itching. He has Crohn's disease which is well managed with azathioprine. On examination, he is jaundiced with hepatomegaly. LFTs show a raised ALP, conjugated bilirubin and γ-GT. A non-invasive liver screen is positive for P-ANCA.

14) A 42-year-old female presents to her primary care doctor with a 3-day history of jaundice following a respiratory tract infection. LFTs show raised unconjugated bilirubin. Her doctor arranges several tests but 2 days following the consultation the patient contacts her doctor informing them the jaundice has resolved.

15) An 18-year-old male presents to the emergency department with abdominal pain, priapism, fatigue, headache and shortness of breath. On examination, he is visibly jaundiced, tachycardic and tachypnoeic, and symmetrical painful swelling in the hands is noted. LFTs show a raised unconjugated bilirubin.

## Small bowel disease

| | | | |
|---|---|---|---|
| a. | Tropical sprue. | e. | Gastrointestinal stromal tumours. |
| b. | Coeliac disease. | f. | Lactose intolerance. |
| c. | Bacterial gastroenteritis. | g. | Carcinoid tumour. |
| d. | Whipple's disease. | h. | Viral gastroenteritis. |

Match the description of the patient with the most likely diagnosis.

16) An 18-year-old male has a 24-hour history of abdominal pain, watery diarrhoea and vomiting. It initially started following a visit to a new restaurant on the high street. The following day the patient feels better and the diarrhoea has resolved.

17) A 26-year-old female attends her primary care doctor with a 2-month history of abdominal bloating, diarrhoea and weight loss. On examination, she has angular stomatitis and a pruritic vesicular rash on her elbows. She has a past medical history of Type 1 diabetes.

18) A 32-year-old male is admitted to the emergency department with abdominal pain, distention, joint pain and vomiting. On examination, he is pyrexial at 38.2°C and has lymphadenopathy. Endoscopic biopsies show PAS-positive macrophages in the lamina propria containing Gram-positive bacilli.

19) A 26-year-old female presents to her primary care doctor as she is embarrassed following several episodes of flatulence, bloating, diarrhoea and rumbling noises in her stomach which occurs following the ingestion of dairy products.

20) A 42-year-old male presents to the emergency department with a 24-hour history of profuse diarrhoea. On examination, he is flushed, hypotensive and has a mild wheeze. He has had right upper quadrant pain for the past 3 months with a 2-stone weight loss but did not attend his primary care doctor as he did not have time.

## Gastric pathology

| | | | |
|---|---|---|---|
| a. | Oral ferrous sulfate. | e. | Partial gastrectomy. |
| b. | Vitamin B$_{12}$ injection. | f. | Gastric bypass. |
| c. | Proton pump inhibitors. | g. | Oral glucocorticoids. |
| d. | *H. pylori* eradication therapy. | h. | Metoclopramide. |

Match the description of the patient with the most appropriate treatment option.

21) A 42-year-old male presents to the emergency department following two episodes of haematemesis. He is tachycardic and hypotensive. He is resuscitated and transferred for immediate endoscopy which locates a bleeding gastric ulcer and is treated with adrenaline. The patient is transferred to the gastroenterology ward but 24 hours later has another haemorrhagic episode which is worse in nature.

22) A 42-year-old male presents to her primary care doctor with a 3-month history of dyspepsia and intermittent epigastric pain that occurs after food. He has noticed recently that he has a dry cough in the morning. He denies any weight loss. Blood results are unremarkable.

23) A 26-year-old male presents to the emergency department with epigastric pain following food. He is otherwise well. He is discharged and given an appointment for an outpatient endoscopy which shows inflammation of the stomach mucosa. The *Campylobacter*-like organism (CLO) test is positive.

24) A 68-year-old male presents to his primary care doctor with a 6-week history of fatigue, pallor and shortness of breath. A full blood count shows a megaloblastic macrocytic anaemia.

25) A 25-year-old male attends the emergency department from his primary care doctor with a 1-month history of abdominal pain, diarrhoea and weight loss. The symptoms have increased in frequency over the past 24 hours and on examination, he has a fever, right iliac fossa tenderness and several aphthous ulcers. Bloods show a raised CRP and platelets. He is usually fit and well with no past medical history.

## Colorectal disease

| | | | |
|---|---|---|---|
| a. | Irritable bowel syndrome. | e. | Acute diverticulitis. |
| b. | Crohn's disease. | f. | Pseudomembranous colitis. |
| c. | Ulcerative colitis. | g. | Chronic constipation. |
| d. | Ischaemic colitis. | h. | Haemorrhoids. |

Match the description of the patient with the most likely diagnosis.

26) A 65-year-old female presents to her primary care doctor with a 24-hour history of abdominal pain and intermittent rectal bleeding. On examination, she has mild tenderness in the left iliac fossa and has a mild fever.

27) A 28-year-old intravenous drug user is admitted for a cellulitis. He is treated with IV antibiotics; however, 3 days after commencing antibiotics he develops a fever, tachycardia and profuse bloody diarrhoea. He informs the medical team he has had three courses of antibiotics in the past 2 months.

28) A 36-year-old male presents to his primary care doctor with a 5-month history of intermittent abdominal pain, bloating and constipation; symptoms are usually relieved by defecation. The patient denies any weight loss and blood tests are all unremarkable.

29) A 70-year-old male with known ischaemic heart disease is admitted with a 6-hour history of severe left iliac fossa pain with several episodes of bloody diarrhoea. Blood tests reveal a raised WCC and raised lactate. Abdominal X-ray shows thumb printing of the descending colon.

30) A 24-year old female presents to her primary care doctor with a 2-week history of bloody diarrhoea and mucus. She is opening her bowels 8-10 times per day. She has noticed crampy lower abdominal pain. On examination, she is tender in the left iliac fossa. Bloods show a raised CRP and WCC.

## Hepatobiliary disease

a.   Acute cholecystitis.                     e.   Hepatocellular carcinoma.
b.   Primary sclerosing cholangitis.   f.   Liver failure.
c.   Cholangiocarcinoma.                  g.   Haemochromatosis.
d.   Primary biliary cirrhosis.            h.   Drug-induced liver injury.

Match the description of the patient with the most likely diagnosis.

31) A 42-year-old female presents to her primary care doctor with abdominal pain, fatigue and pruritis. She reports paler stools and dark urine. On examination, she has right upper quadrant pain with hepatomegaly and jaundice. Blood results show a raised ALP, γ-GT and a positive anti-mitochondrial antibody.

32) A 52-year-old male is referred to the gastroenterology clinic with a 2-week history of sudden-onset jaundice. He is known to have AF, ischaemic heart disease and Type 2 diabetes. He currently takes amiodarone, ramipril and gliclazide. Bloods show a raised ALT but normal ALP.

33) A 65-year-old female with known primary sclerosing cholangitis presents to the gastroenterology clinic with a 2-month history of weight loss and jaundice. On examination, she has abdominal distention, shifting dullness and right upper quadrant abdominal pain. Bloods reveal an elevated α-fetoprotein.

34) A 48-year-old male attends the gastroenterology clinic with an 8-week history of right upper quadrant pain, fatigue, weight loss and itching. He is known to have HIV. On examination, he is jaundiced with hepatomegaly. LFTs show a raised ALP, conjugated bilirubin and γ-GT and positive P-ANCA.

35) A 48-year-old known alcoholic presents to the emergency department with a 5-day history of nausea, anorexia and fatigue. The doctor assessing him believes the patient is confused and is unable to recall events or familiar surroundings. On examination, the patient has jaundice and signs of chronic alcohol liver disease.

## Pancreatic pathology

a.  Acute pancreatitis.
b.  Zollinger-Ellison syndrome.
c.  Carcinoma head of the pancreas.
d.  Exocrine pancreatic insufficiency.
e.  Pancreatic divisum.
f.  Chronic pancreatitis.
g.  MEN Type 1.
h.  MEN Type 2A.

Match the description of the patient with the most likely diagnosis.

36) A 30-year-old female attends the gastroenterology clinic for review following diagnosis of a pancreatic tumour with a concurrent pituitary adenoma. She is found to have a genetic mutation which predisposes her to these neoplastic lesions.

37) A 38-year-old builder has been reviewed by his primary care doctor for the past 6 months for recurrent dyspepsia. He has tried antacids and high-dose omeprazole with little relief. He undergoes an oesophago-gastroduodenoscopy which show multiple duodenal ulcers. Blood tests note a raised serum gastrin.

38) A 12-year-old male with cystic fibrosis attends the gastroenterology clinic. The medical student in the clinic takes a thorough history and notes he is taking Creon®. The consultant asks the medical student why the patient would be taking this medication.

39) A 42-year old male presents to the emergency department with a 24-hour history of severe epigastric pain radiating to the back. He has a past medical history of gallstones. On examination, he is tender in the epigastrium and blood results show an amylase of 2800IU/L.

40) A 72-year-old male presents with a 6-month history of painless jaundice, anorexia, weight loss and epigastric pain. He has pale stools and dark urine. He has a history of chronic pancreatitis. On examination, the gallbladder is palpable but non-tender. He has multiple transient swellings and redness of limb veins. Blood results show a normocytic anaemia with a raised CA19-9.

## Hepatitis

a.  Hepatitis A.                     e.  Hepatitis E.
b.  Hepatitis B.                     f.  Alcohol-induced hepatitis.
c.  Hepatitis C.                     g.  Autoimmune hepatitis.
d.  Hepatitis D.                     h.  Viral hepatitis.

Match the description of the patient with the most likely diagnosis.

41)  A 30-year-old female with known coeliac disease presents with mild jaundice. On examination, she is visibly jaundiced but no other pathology is noted. She denies alcohol or drug use. Blood tests show a raised AST and ALT, and are positive for both anti-nuclear and anti-smooth muscle antibodies.

42)  An 18-year-old backpacker returns from travelling around Thailand and experiences yellowing of his skin and diarrhoea. His stools appear paler and urine darker than usual. He indulged in a shellfish meal prior to completing his trip.

43)  A 34-year-old Moroccan female presents with fatigue and itchy skin. She is a known intravenous drug user. On examination, she is clinically jaundiced.

44)  A 26-year-old intravenous drug user with known hepatitis B attends the emergency department with jaundice. He undergoes several investigations on the gastroenterology ward and the medical team inform him he has a second form of hepatitis that only causes disease in those already infected with hepatitis B.

45)  A 42-year-old homeless male attends the emergency department with abdominal pain. He admits to drinking 20 units of alcohol per day. On examination, he has right upper quadrant tenderness, hepatomegaly and mild ascites. Blood results show deranged liver function tests.

## Short answer questions

1) A 22-year-old female presents to the emergency department 24 hours after a paracetamol overdose. The doctor assessing her believes the patient is confused. On examination, the patient is jaundiced. Bloods reveal deranged LFTs and a coagulopathy.

   a. What is the underlying diagnosis? 1 mark
   b. Give four other symptoms of this condition. 2 marks
   c. Give four other signs of this condition. 2 marks
   d. Name two possible treatments for this condition. 2 marks
   e. State three complications of this condition. 3 marks

2) A 38-year-old female presents to her primary care doctor with a 3-month history of dyspepsia and intermittent epigastric pain that occurs after food. She has noticed recently that she has a dry cough in the morning. She denies any weight loss. The doctor treats her for gastro-oesophageal reflux disease (GORD).

   a. Name four risk factors for GORD. 2 marks
   b. Give four appropriate investigations for this condition. 2 marks
   c. Define four factors requiring urgent upper GI investigation. 2 marks
   d. Describe four possible treatment options in this patient. 2 marks
   e. Name four possible complications of GORD. 2 marks

3) A 68-year-old female is admitted to the emergency department with a 2-day history of painless jaundice. She believes she has lost 2 stone in weight over the past 4 weeks. On examination, she is jaundiced with a palpable gallbladder and palpable mass in the epigastrium. The doctor believes she has an obstructive jaundice.

a.  How is jaundice classified and provide two examples for each?   3 marks
b.  When is jaundice clinically detectable?                         1 mark
c.  Describe urine and stool findings for obstructive jaundice.     1 mark
d.  Name four components of a non-invasive liver screen.            2 marks
e.  Name three complications of jaundice.                           3 marks

4) A 50-year-old alcoholic male is brought into the emergency department by an ambulance crew following a fall in the street. He has fractured his right femur and requires admission to the orthopaedic ward. It is noted that a liver biopsy taken 6 months ago showed Mallory's hyaline. The patient admits to drinking 3L of cider per day for the past 18 months.

a.  What is Mallory's hyaline?                                      1 mark
b.  Define the stages of liver damage from normal to cirrhosis.    3 marks
c.  Name two medications used to prevent alcohol withdrawal.       2 marks
d.  What are the indications for liver transplant in alcohol-related liver   1 mark
    disease?
e.  Specify three complications of chronic alcohol consumption.     3 marks

5) A 42-year-old Somali migrant is seen by his primary care doctor for a 10-day history of right upper quadrant pain and jaundice. He has recently returned from Somalia visiting his family. He has noted paler stools and darker urine for the past 2 weeks. On examination, he is visibly jaundiced. His blood results show deranged LFTs and a positive anti-HBc IgM, positive HBsAg, positive HBeAg, a high viral load, negative HBeAb, negative anti-HBc IgG and negative HBsAb in keeping with acute hepatitis B infection.

a. Name four risk factors for this condition. 4 marks
b. Name two treatment options for this patient. 2 marks
c. Give two complications of hepatitis B infection. 2 marks
d. What would the serological profile be for a patient vaccinated against hepatitis B? 1 mark
e. What form of hepatitis requires co-infection with hepatitis B? 1 mark

6) A 26-year-old female presents to her primary care doctor with a 3-week history of bloody diarrhoea and mucus. She is opening her bowels nine times per day. She has noticed crampy lower abdominal pain. On examination, she is tender in the left iliac fossa. Bloods show a raised CRP and WCC.

a. Name three factors to assess the severity of ulcerative colitis. 3 marks
b. List four differences between ulcerative colitis and Crohn's disease. 4 marks
c. Specify two extra-intestinal features of Crohn's disease. 1 mark
d. Name two complications of ulcerative colitis. 1 mark
e. Give two complications of Crohn's disease. 1 mark

7) A 24-year-old female presents to the emergency department 4 hours after ingesting 28 x 500mg paracetamol tablets. She informs the staff that this was a suicide attempt as she has recently split up with her boyfriend. On examination, she appears well.

a. How should the patient be assessed? 1 mark
b. List three questions to assess the seriousness of the attempt. 3 marks
c. Name two investigations other than paracetamol levels that should be requested. 2 marks
d. When the paracetamol level returns what is used to assess whether treatment is required? 1 mark
e. Name three management options for a paracetamol overdose with no evidence of hepatic or renal failure. 3 marks

8) A 32-year-old female presents to her primary care doctor with a 5-month history of intermittent abdominal pain, bloating and constipation. Symptoms are usually relieved by defecation.

a. What is the underlying diagnosis? 1 mark
b. What is usually found when investigating this condition? 1 mark
c. Describe the Rome III criteria for this condition. 4 marks
d. Name four management options for this condition. 2 marks
e. Name two psychiatric conditions associated with this diagnosis. 2 marks

9) A 22-year-old medical student is due to attend a clinical placement on gastroenterology; however, prior to leaving the house he has an episode of diarrhoea which is non-bloody and vomiting. He diagnoses himself with acute gastroenteritis and decides it is appropriate to stay at home.

a. Name four bacteria that can cause acute diarrhoea. 4 marks
b. Name two viruses that can cause acute diarrhoea. 2 marks
c. Provide two treatments that would be appropriate. 1 mark
d. Define four infection control measures that should be commenced. 2 marks
e. If he has had a recent course of antibiotics, what condition should you be concerned about? 1 mark

10) A 48-year-old female presents to the gastroenterology unit with a 4-month history of dyspepsia and epigastric pain after food. She denies any weight loss, dysphagia or vomiting. The consultant refers her for an OGD. He believes she may have Barrett's oesophagus or a peptic ulcer.

a. Name two other causes of dyspepsia. 1 mark
b. Give six red flag symptoms for dyspepsia. 3 marks
c. What would a biopsy show with Barrett's oesophagus? 1 mark
d. Name three tests that can be used to test for *H. pylori*. 3 marks
e. Name the two components of *H. pylori* eradication therapy. 2 marks

11) An 82-year-old female is admitted to the care of the elderly ward following a fall at home. She appears malnourished. The dietician recommends artificial feeding and the consultant in charge asks his team to ensure daily bloods are performed if artificial feeding is commenced.

| | | |
|---|---|---|
| a. | What condition is monitored for when restarting feeding? | 1 mark |
| b. | What tool can be used to screen for malnutrition? | 1 mark |
| c. | Name six risk factors for malnutrition in adults. | 3 marks |
| d. | Specify daily requirements for glucose, protein, sodium, water, potassium and chloride. | 3 marks |
| e. | State two management options to improve the patient's nutrition. | 2 marks |

12) A 25-year-old female presents with a 3-month history of diarrhoea, bloating and malaise. On examination, she is pale with angular stomatitis.

| | | |
|---|---|---|
| a. | List six causes of chronic diarrhoea in adults. | 3 marks |
| b. | Give four investigations that can be considered in this patient. | 2 marks |
| c. | If the patient had a positive tissue transglutaminase what would be the underlying diagnosis? | 1 mark |
| d. | State two treatment options for the patient in question c. | 2 marks |
| e. | Name two complications of this condition in question c. | 2 marks |

13) A 42-year-old male is admitted to the emergency department with a 4-hour history of haematemesis. He has had four episodes of vomiting blood. On examination, he is tachycardic and hypotensive. The doctor assessing the patient suspects the patient is having an upper GI bleed.

a.  How would you assess this patient?                           1 mark
b.  Name four common causes of an upper GI bleed.               2 marks
c.  State three investigations for this patient.                 3 marks
d.  Give three treatment options for this patient.              3 marks
e.  Name the scoring system that can be used to predict the need for  1 mark
    clinical intervention in patients with an upper GI bleed.

# Chapter 4

# Renal

## QUESTIONS

### Single best answer questions

1) Furosemide increases diuresis by inhibiting the co-transport of $Na^+/K^+/2Cl^-$ in which part of the nephron?

a. Thick ascending loop of Henle.
b. Thin ascending loop of Henle.
c. Collecting duct.
d. Proximal tubule.

2) Which part of the nephron is responsible for the majority of sodium resorption?

a. Cortical collecting duct.
b. Thin ascending loop of Henle.
c. Proximal convoluted tubule.
d. Thick ascending loop of Henle.

3) Which of the following treatments is an appropriate first-line antibiotic for uncomplicated urinary tract infection in a 27-year-old female?

a. Co-amoxiclav.
b. Gentamicin.
c. Fosfomycin.
d. Nitrofurantoin.

4) A 26-year-old male presents with haematuria. He reports a recent viral illness and sore throat but is otherwise well. What is the diagnosis?

a. IgA nephropathy.
b. Anti-GBM disease.
c. Proliferative glomerulonephritis.
d. SLE.

5) A patient is diagnosed with anti-GBM disease following a renal biopsy. Which other organ is commonly affected by the condition?

a. Liver.
b. Brain.
c. Skin.
d. Lung.

6) Anti-GBM disease involves auto-antibody production to which type of collagen?

a. Type I.
b. Type II.
c. Type III.
d. Type IV.

7) IgA nephropathy is what kind of hypersensitivity reaction?

a. Type I.
b. Type II.
c. Type III.
d. Type IV.

8) Established renal failure is diagnosed at what glomerular filtration rate?

a. Less than 10ml/min.
b. Less than 15ml/min.
c. Less than 20ml/min.
d. Less than 25ml/min.

9) Under what main mechanism does haemodialysis occur to remove waste products such as uric acid?

a. Ultrafiltration.
b. Diffusion.
c. Osmosis.
d. Active transport.

10) What main group of organisms is responsible for the majority of peritoneal dialysis-associated peritonitis?

a. *Staphylococcus*.
b. Fungi.
c. Gram-negative organisms.
d. *Streptococcus*.

11) Which of the following analgesics is a recognised nephrotoxin?

a. Paracetamol.
b. Fentanyl.
c. Ibuprofen.
d. Codeine.

12) Which syndrome is associated with sensorineural deafness, renal insufficiency and lenticonus?

a. Alport's syndrome.
b. Ramsay-Hunt syndrome.
c. Fanconi syndrome.
d. Gilbert's syndrome.

13) Polycystic kidney disease is primarily transmitted by which mode of inheritance?

a) X-linked dominant.
b) X-linked recessive.
c) Autosomal dominant.
d) Autosomal recessive.

14) A 3-year-old child develops an acute illness associated with diarrhoea and vomiting which is later confirmed as *E. coli*. Three weeks later they present to the emergency department after their father reports another episode of severe bloody diarrhoea. What associated complication have they developed?

a. Henoch-Schönlein purpura.
b. Haemolytic uraemic syndrome.
c. Disseminated intravascular coagulopathy.
d. Thrombotic thrombocytopenic purpura.

15) A 4-year-old boy presents to primary care with a low-grade fever and is generally unwell. On examination, you feel a mass and suspect a tumour. What is the most common renal neoplasm in children?

a. Wilms' tumour.
b. Renal cell carcinoma.
c. Transitional cell carcinoma.
d. Leiomyosarcoma.

16) A 56-year-old male patient who has a history of smoking is diagnosed with renal cell carcinoma after investigation for microscopic haematuria. Which of the following is the least likely site for metastases to occur?

a. Liver.
b. Spleen.
c. Lung.
d. Bone.

17) A 37-year-old female presents to her primary care doctor with episodes of haematuria, coughing up blood, a sense of malaise and is lethargic. On examination, you notice she has mouth ulcers and looks systemically unwell with a purple, non-blanching rash on her legs. What is the most likely diagnosis?

a.   IgA nephropathy.
b.   Anti-GBM disease.
c.   Granulomatosis with polyangiitis.
d.   Meningococcal septicaemia.

18) A 24-year-old male patient attends the emergency department with frank haematuria. He is otherwise fit and well, but does report a recent illness with a painful and sore throat 3 weeks ago. What is the most likely diagnosis?

a.   IgA nephropathy.
b.   Focal segmental glomerulosclerosis.
c.   Post-infective glomerulonephritis.
d.   Anti-GBM disease.

19) What three features are commonly seen in nephritic syndrome?

a.   Haematuria, hypotension and proteinuria.
b.   Haematuria, hypertension and proteinuria.
c.   Haematuria, polyuria and proteinuria.
d.   Oedema, hypoalbuminaemia and hyperlipidaemia.

20) What is the normal urine output for an adult?

a.  0.25-0.5ml/kg/hour.
b.  2-3ml/kg/hour.
c.  0.5-1ml/kg/hour.
d.  0.1-0.5ml/kg/hour.

21) What is the normal urine output for a child?

a.  0.25-1ml/kg/hour.
b.  1-2ml/kg/hour.
c.  0.5-1.5ml/kg/hour.
d.  2-3ml/kg/hour.

22) The hospital laboratory technician bleeps you to inform you that one of your ward patients has a hyperkalaemia of 6.95mmol/L. You urgently review the patient who looks very unwell with an ECG showing wide QRS complexes. What medication would you administer urgently to stabilise the myocardium?

a.  5mg of nebulised salbutamol.
b.  1L of 0.9% NaCl IV STAT.
c.  IV insulin with glucose.
d.  10ml of 10% calcium gluconate.

23) Which antibiotic must be dose reduced in chronic kidney disease with an eGFR 29ml/min?

a.  Gentamycin.
b.  Amoxicillin.
c.  Trimethoprim.
d.  Phenoxymethylpenicillin.

# Extended matching questions

## Acute kidney injury

|     |                                |     |                          |
| --- | ------------------------------ | --- | ------------------------ |
| a.  | Sepsis.                        | e.  | Glomerulonephritis.      |
| b.  | Acute interstitial nephritis.  | f.  | Chronic kidney disease.  |
| c.  | Hypovolaemia.                  | g.  | IgA nephropathy.         |
| d.  | Renal outflow obstruction.     | h.  | Acute tubular necrosis.  |

Match the description with the most likely cause of the acute kidney injury.

1) A 54-year-old male presents with tachycardia, fever and hypotension. He has a history of COPD and a productive cough for 5 days.

2) A 74-year-old male with known Stage 3 chronic kidney disease is commenced on a 2-week course of ibuprofen for a swollen wrist. He presents 10 days later with vomiting, malaise and reduced urine output.

3) A 16-year-old female who has a long-term suprapubic catheter admits she is struggling to manage. On inspection you see debris in the tube and her bladder scan reveals 765ml in the bladder.

4) An 87-year-old female is brought in to see her primary care doctor for review by her carer. She has low mood and reduced oral intake. Routine bloods show a markedly raised urea and an increase in creatinine from baseline.

5) A 45-year-old male with intense loin to groin pain, reduced urine output and microscopic haematuria on urinalysis.

## Interpreting blood test results

| | | | |
|---|---|---|---|
| a. | C-reactive protein. | e. | Creatinine. |
| b. | ESR. | f. | eGFR. |
| c. | WCC. | g. | Urea. |
| d. | Neutrophils. | h. | Potassium. |

Select the most appropriate biochemical marker with the description.

6) Used as a diagnostic marker for acute kidney injury.

7) Used as a diagnostic marker for chronic kidney disease.

8) Classified as raised when greater then 5.5mmol/L

9) The result is affected by race and diet.

10) Often raised in bacterial infections, but also in the presence of malignancy or rheumatological conditions.

## Glomerulonephritis

| | | | |
|---|---|---|---|
| a. | IgA nephropathy. | e. | Minimal change. |
| b. | SLE. | f. | Mesangiocapillary glomerulonephritis. |
| c. | Anti-glomerular basement disease. | g. | Nephrotic syndrome. |
| d. | Post-streptococcal glomerulonephritis. | h. | Nephritic syndrome. |

Match the description with the most likely diagnosis.

11) Characterised by oedema, proteinuria and hypoalbuminaemia. Hyperlipidaemia is often present.

12) Most common cause of nephrotic syndrome in children.

13) Typically presents as haematuria in a young male 2-3 days post-upper respiratory tract infection.

14) Renal biopsy will show large glomeruli with mesangial proliferation and thickened capillary walls giving a 'tramline' appearance.

15) Episodes of haematuria seen in a male patient up to 12 weeks post-throat or skin infection.

## Renal transplantation

a.   Renal cell carcinoma.          e.   Acute rejection.

b.   Cadaveric donor.               f.   Chronic rejection.

c.   Living related donor.          g.   Non-beating donor.

d.   Live unrelated donor.          h.   Organ donation.

## Match the description with the most likely answer.

16)   An absolute contraindication to becoming an organ donor.

17)   Rejection of an organ occurring at 7 months.

18)   Organs are retrieved from a brain-stem dead donor with supported circulation and ventilation.

19)   A 23-year-old female, 3 months post-renal transplantation surgery presents with rising creatinine, fever and pain at the operative site.

20)   The partner of a 45-year-old man with end-stage renal failure wishes to be considered for donation of their kidney.

## Function of the nephron

a.  Bowman's capsule.               e.  Thick ascending limb.
b.  Proximal convoluted tubule.     f.  Thin ascending limb.
c.  Descending loop of Henle.       g.  Distal convoluted tubule.
d.  Collecting duct.                h.  Glomerulus.

## Match the description with one of the above options.

21) The renal corpuscle contains the Bowman's capsule and this other structure.

22) Situated in between the loop of Henle and the collecting ducts.

23) Furosemide inhibits cotransport of $Na^+/K^+/2Cl^-$ at this part of the nephron.

24) The site of action of antidiuretic hormone to increase resorption of water at aquaporin channels.

25) The main site of pathology in diabetic nephropathy.

## The glomerulus

| | | | |
|---|---|---|---|
| a. | Mesangial cells. | e. | Macula densa. |
| b. | Afferent arteriole. | f. | Juxtaglomerular cells. |
| c. | Efferent arteriole. | g. | Podocyte cells. |
| d. | Bowman's capsule. | h. | Glomerular basement membrane. |

## Match the description with the above options.

26) The site of immune complex deposition in Goodpasture's syndrome.

27) The site of blood exiting the glomerulus.

28) Cells that synthesize, store and secrete the enzyme renin.

29) Situated in the distal tubule, these cells are in contact with the glomerulus and are sensitive to sodium chloride concentration.

30) The site of blood entering the glomerulus.

## Hormones and the kidney

| | | | |
|---|---|---|---|
| a. | Renin. | e. | Antidiuretic hormone. |
| b. | Erythropoietin. | f. | Calcitriol. |
| c. | Angiotensin I. | g. | Parathyroid hormone. |
| d. | Angiotensin II. | h. | Atrial natriuretic peptide. |

## Match the description with the most likely hormone.

31) Produced by interstitial cells in the kidney, liver and brain.

32) When baroreceptors detect decreased arterial blood pressure this hormone is produced in the juxtaglomerular apparatus.

33) This hormone acts on venous and arterial smooth muscle cells to cause vasoconstriction.

34) Release of this hormone increases calcium levels by promoting the uptake of calcium from the gut and calcium resorption in the kidney.

35) Its secretion is stimulated by cell hypoxia.

## Pharmacology and the kidney

a. Ramipril.

b. Gentamicin.

c. Metformin.

d. Sitagliptin.

e. Nitrofurantoin.

f. Trimethoprim.

g. Lithium.

h. Amlodipine.

## Match the description with the most likely medication.

36) A common cause of nephrogenic diabetes insipidus.

37) Antihypertensive which must be monitored with U&Es after commencing.

38) Aminoglycoside antibiotic which must be reduced in chronic kidney disease.

39) Temporary cessation of this medication used to treat diabetes is advised during acute kidney injury.

40) Folic acid inhibitor used to treat urinary tract infection.

## Urine microscopy

a.   Cystine crystals.                    e.   White blood cell casts.
b.   Calcium oxalate crystals.            f.   Waxy casts.
c.   Red blood cell casts.                g.   Hyaline casts.
d.   Uric acid crystals.                  h.   Granular casts.

## Match the description with the most likely answer.

41)   May be found in normal individuals in the presence of fever, dehydration or exercise.

42)   Often a positive finding in nephritic syndrome.

43)   Indicates infection or inflammation.

44)   The presence of these in fresh urine indicates an increased risk of renal calculi.

45)   Seen in longstanding kidney disease.

# Short answer questions

1) A 34-year-old female presents to the emergency department severely lethargic and oliguric. Her husband states that her family have kidney problems. On examination, she is hypertensive and complains of abdominal and back pain. The attending doctor suspects a diagnosis of polycystic kidney disease.

| | | |
|---|---|---|
| a. | Give two other causes of nephrogenic hypertension. | 2 marks |
| b. | Name two modes of inheritance in polycystic kidney disease. | 2 marks |
| c. | Name two extrarenal manifestations of this condition. | 2 marks |
| d. | Above what blood pressure values indicate hypertension? | 2 marks |
| e. | Explain why kidney stones occur in this condition. | 2 marks |

2) A 45-year-old female attends her primary care doctor complaining of headaches. The attending doctor diagnoses her with hypertension and initiates treatment with ramipril. After 2 weeks, the U&Es are checked and her eGFR has dropped from 87ml/min to 43ml/min.

| | | |
|---|---|---|
| a. | What class of drug is ramipril? | 1 mark |
| b. | Name two common side effects of ramipril. | 2 marks |
| c. | What condition may have caused the decrease in eGFR? | 1 mark |
| d. | Name the four variables used to calculate the eGFR. | 4 marks |
| e. | Name two factors which may affect the accuracy of the eGFR. | 2 marks |

3) A 67-year-old male presents to his primary care doctor with a first episode of haematuria. He is concerned that he may have cancer.

a.  What is the most common type of kidney cancer in the UK?  1 mark

b.  Which part of the nephron does this cancer affect?  1 mark

c.  Specify one other finding on abdominal examination.  1 mark

d.  Give four other risk factors for this condition.  4 marks

e.  Give three other non-neoplastic causes of frank haematuria.  3 marks

4)  A 43-year-old female is admitted to the acute medical unit with urinary sepsis. The nurse informs you that despite catheterisation, the patient's urine output is poor. You suspect a diagnosis of acute kidney injury (AKI).

a.  Give two diagnostic markers of AKI.  4 marks

b.  Name one class of drugs which may precipitate AKI.  1 marks

c.  Name two physiological parameters you will need to monitor in a patient with AKI.  2 marks

d.  Name two biochemical parameters you will need to monitor in a patient with AKI.  2 marks

e.  The patient weighs 75kg. Calculate the minimum expected urine output over 24 hours for this patient.  1 mark

5)  A 36-year-old male presents to the emergency department with a 2-week history of increasing lethargy, nausea and vomiting. He tells you he is a Type 1 diabetic and has "bad" kidneys. His blood glucose is 5.3mmol/L.

a.  Give an appropriate intravenous fluid you may use to rehydrate the patient.  1 mark

b.  Give four indications for acute dialysis.  4 marks

c.  His eGFR is 17ml/min. What stage of chronic kidney disease does he have?  1 mark

d.  Other than glycosuria, what will be present on urinalysis?  1 mark

e.  Give three treatments for end-stage renal failure.  3 marks

6) A patient with end-stage renal failure on haemodialysis three times a week presents with low mood. He is tearful and wants to commit suicide as he cannot cope with his illness.

| | | |
|---|---|---|
| a. | Give four symptoms of chronic renal failure. | 4 marks |
| b. | Give one diagnostic feature of depression. | 1 mark |
| c. | Give two complications associated with haemodialysis. | 2 marks |
| d. | Give two complications associated with peritoneal dialysis. | 2 marks |
| e. | How could you assess the severity of their depression? | 1 mark |

7) You are the junior medical doctor on call. You receive a referral from a primary care doctor who tells you they are sending in a 61-year-old male with chronic kidney disease Stage III and a hyperkalaemia of 7.2mmol/L. On admission, you request an urgent ECG which shows features of hyperkalaemia.

| | | |
|---|---|---|
| a. | Name three ECG findings of hyperkalaemia. | 3 marks |
| b. | Give three immediate treatments for hyperkalaemia. | 3 marks |
| c. | Give two causes of hyperkalaemia other than renal failure. | 2 marks |
| d. | Name one hormone which increases renal potassium excretion. | 1 mark |
| e. | In which organ is this hormone synthesized? | 1 mark |

8) An 8-year-old child presents to the emergency department with swelling of their legs, malaise and fatigue. You suspect a diagnosis of nephrotic syndrome.

| | | |
|---|---|---|
| a. | Name one bedside test that can confirm your suspicions. | 1 mark |
| b. | Give the three diagnostic features of nephrotic syndrome. | 3 marks |
| c. | Name the commonest cause of this condition in children. | 1 mark |
| d. | What is the mainstay of treatment of the above disease? | 1 mark |
| e. | Give four other causes of primary nephrotic syndrome. | 4 marks |

9) A 21-year-old female presents with symptoms of fever, pain on passing urine and frequent urination for 2 days. The patient informs you she is 8/40 weeks' pregnant.

a. Give the most common causative organism for urinary tract infection (UTI) in young women in the community.    1 mark

b. Give two features of UTI on urine dipstick.    2 marks

c. Which first-line antibiotic commonly used to treat uncomplicated UTI must be avoided in this patient and why?    2 marks

d. What is the definition of a complicated UTI?    1 mark

e. Give four risk factors for UTI.    4 marks

10) A 19-year-old male presents to the emergency department with his third episode of visible haematuria. He is usually fit and well but does mention a recent sore throat last week. You suspect this is a glomerulonephritis condition.

a. Considering the history, what is the most likely diagnosis and give two other clinical features?    3 marks

b. Describe the pathophysiology of the condition.    2 marks

c. Give two treatments of the condition.    2 marks

d. What type of hypersensitivity reaction is this?    1 mark

e. Give two conditions which present with nephritic syndrome.    2 marks

11) A 27-year-old male presents with haemoptysis. He admits to smoking 20 cigarettes a day. You organise a chest X-ray and some routine bloods. As he is leaving the consultation room, he also mentions that he has noticed blood occasionally in his urine for the past 6 weeks.

a.  What diagnosis do you suspect?                                           1 mark
b.  Describe the pathophysiology of the condition.                          3 marks
c.  Give three treatments for this condition.                               3 marks
d.  What test is required to confirm renal involvement?                      1 mark
e.  Give two systemic features of this condition.                          2 marks

12) A patient is commenced on haemodialysis for end-stage renal failure secondary to Type 2 diabetes mellitus. During their first session they begin to feel sick complaining of a headache. Thirty minutes later they start to vomit and become drowsy.

a.  What syndrome is the above and what causes this?                        2 marks
b.  Name two other potential complications of haemodialysis.               2 marks
c.  Briefly describe the process of haemodialysis.                          3 marks
d.  Give two dietary modifications recommended for patients with           2 marks
    chronic kidney disease.
e.  Name one common cause of anaemia in patients with chronic kidney        1 mark
    disease.

13) An 87-year-old female is brought in by ambulance after being found on the floor by her carers. She tells you that unfortunately she was on the floor for at least 18 hours unable to get up. Her past medical history reveals only severe osteoarthritis in her hips. Her initial bloods are shown below.

| | |
|---|---|
| eGFR | 23ml/min |
| Creatinine | 187μmol/L |
| Urea | 14mmol/L |
| Creatinine kinase | 4523 IU/L |
| CRP | <1mg/L |

a.  By what mechanism has the creatinine kinase risen?  1 mark
b.  Give two causes of AKI given the history and blood results.  2 marks
c.  Which other important condition is associated with a rise in CK, and  2 marks
    name one bedside test you could perform?
d.  Specify four other causes of a raised CK.  4 marks
e.  What is the mainstay of treatment for AKI in this case?  1 mark

# Chapter 5

# Endocrinology
## QUESTIONS

## Single best answer questions

1) Which is the most common gene association in Type 1 diabetes?

a. TCF7L2.
b. HLD-DR3/4.
c. SLC30A8.
d. HNF4A.

2) What is the correct value for diagnosing diabetes using fasting glucose?

a. <7.0mmol/L.
b. >6.0mmol/L.
c. >7.0mmol/L.
d. >6.5mmol/L.

3) Which of the following is the most appropriate management of a hyperosmolar hyperglycaemic state?

a.   Antibiotic therapy.
b.   Rapid IV fluids and insulin.
c.   Slow IV fluids and insulin.
d.   10% dextrose IV.

4) Which of the following constitutes a major aspect of managing DKA?

a.   Fixed-rate insulin infusion.
b.   Variable-rate insulin infusion.
c.   Stat doses of NovoRapid®.
d.   Immediate antibiotic therapy.

5) What is the initial management for hypoglycaemia, in a patient who is conscious but slightly drowsy?

a.   Glucagon IM 1mg.
b.   50ml 20% dextrose IV.
c.   20-30mg fast-acting carbohydrate (e.g. glucose oral gel).
d.   Slow-release carbohydrate (e.g. toast).

6) Which of the following is most indicative of Graves' disease?

a.   Pre-tibial myxoedema.
b.   Anxiety.
c.   Palmar erythema.
d.   Hair loss.

7) What is the most common cause of hypothyroidism worldwide?

a. Hashimoto's thyroiditis.
b. Iodine deficiency.
c. Congenital.
d. Lithium therapy.

8) Which results would you expect most often in hypothyroidism?

a. Low T3, low T4, raised TSH.
b. Raised T3, low T4, raised TSH.
c. Raised T3, raised T4, low TSH.
d. Low T3, low T4, low TSH.

9) Which of the following results would you expect to see in someone with primary hyperparathyroidism?

a. Low PTH, low calcium, high phosphate.
b. Raised PTH, raised calcium, low phosphate.
c. Raised PTH, low calcium, low phosphate.
d. Raised PTH, raised calcium, raised phosphate.

10) Which is the most appropriate first step in managing hypercalcaemia?

a. IV bisphosphonate.
b. IV fluid resuscitation.
c. Bone protection.
d. Haemodialysis.

11) Which of the following is the most appropriate initial management of someone with mild hypoparathyroidism?

a. Vitamin D and calcium supplements.
b. IV calcium gluconate.
c. IV bisphosphonate.
d. IV fluid resuscitation.

12) Which of the following best describes Cushing's disease?

a. Ectopic ACTH secretion.
b. Adrenal adenoma.
c. Adrenal carcinoma.
d. Pituitary adenoma secreting ACTH.

13) Which of the following would you see in Cushing's syndrome?

a. Low-dose dexamethasone test → low cortisol;
   High-dose dexamethasone test → low cortisol.
b. Low-dose dexamethasone test → no change;
   High-dose dexamethasone test → low cortisol.
c. Low-dose dexamethasone test → no change;
   High-dose dexamethasone test → no change.
d. Low-dose dexamethasone test → high cortisol;
   High-dose dexamethasone test → high cortisol

14) Which of the following is the most common cause of Addison's disease?

a. Sarcoidosis.
b. Adrenalectomy.
c. HIV infection.
d. Autoimmune disease.

15) What is the most appropriate treatment for Addison's disease?

a. Hydrocortisone and fludrocortisone.
b. Hydrocortisone only.
c. Fludrocortisone only.
d. Prednisolone and hydrocortisone.

16) Which of these is not a physiological cause of hyperprolactinaemia?

a. Stress.
b. Breast feeding.
c. Pregnancy.
d. Weight gain.

17) Which of the following is the definitive treatment option for someone with acromegaly as a result of a benign pituitary adenoma?

a. Somatostatin analogue.
b. Dopamine agonists.
c. Trans-sphenoidal surgery.
d. GH receptor antagonists.

18) Which one of the following is correct for a phaeochromocytoma?

a. 50% are extra-adrenal.
b. 10% are bilateral.
c. 90% are malignant.
d. 45% are familial.

19) Which of the following is the most common cause of congenital adrenal hyperplasia?

a. 21-alpha-hydroxylase deficiency.
b. 11-beta-hydroxylase deficiency.
c. Aldosterone synthetase deficiency.
d. 17-alpha-hydroxylase deficiency.

20) A monoclonal tumour of which cell type will cause increased growth hormone secretion?

a. Corticotrophs.
b. Gonadotrophs.
c. Comatotrophs.
d. Thyrotrophs.

21) Which of the following best describes central diabetes insipidus?

a. Failure of the posterior pituitary to produce ADH.
b. Failure of the kidneys to respond to ADH.
c. Excess secretion of ADH from the posterior pituitary.
d. Excess excretion of ADH from the kidneys.

22) Which of the following is the most appropriate first step in treating the syndrome of inappropriate ADH?

a. Hydrocortisone therapy.
b. Fluid restriction.
c. IV fluid resuscitation.
d. Hypertonic saline administration.

23) A possible complication of treating SIADH is central pontine myelinolysis as a result of rapid correction of an electrolyte. Which electrolyte should be closely monitored to avoid this?

a.   Potassium.
b.   Calcium.
c.   Magnesium.
d.   Sodium.

# Extended matching questions

## Diabetes mellitus

a. Type 1 diabetes.
b. Type 2 diabetes.
c. HHS.
d. Diabetic ketoacidosis.

e. Hypoglycaemia — alcohol.
f. Hypoglycaemia — infection.
g. Insulin overdose.
h. Reduced oral intake.

Match the following presentation to the most likely diagnosis.

1) A 75-year-old male presents with a 4-day history of dysuria and urinary frequency. He has experienced several shaking episodes over the last 3 hours. As he is waiting to be assessed he becomes drowsy and his GCS is 13.

2) A 16-year-old female presents to her primary care doctor complaining of frequent urination for the past 2 months. She mentions she feels thirsty and is eating more than normal but still losing weight.

3) A 65-year-old male is found unconscious at home. He has a past medical history of dementia and insulin-dependent Type 2 diabetes. He is found by his carer with a partially emptied medication dispensing system and a half-full insulin injection pen.

4) A 19-year-old male presents to the emergency department with vomiting and abdominal pain. His girlfriend mentions he has lost a lot of weight recently and has been going to the toilet much more than normal. The patient looks dehydrated and on examination you notice a sweet smell to his breath.

5) A 50-year-old female presents to her primary care doctor complaining of thrush-like symptoms, which has occurred multiple times over the last 2 months. She has noticed increased thirst and urinary frequency for the past 2 weeks.

## Drugs used in diabetes

| | | | |
|---|---|---|---|
| a. | Metformin. | e. | Aspirin. |
| b. | Gliclazide. | f. | Ramipril. |
| c. | Rosiglitazone. | g. | Beta-blockers. |
| d. | Acarbose. | h. | Warfarin. |

Match the following side effect with the most likely causative agent.

6) Hypoglycaemia.

7) Nausea.

8) Flatulence.

9) Weight gain.

10) Deranged LFTs.

## Thyroid pathology

| | | | |
|---|---|---|---|
| a. | Graves' disease. | e. | Hashimoto's thyroiditis. |
| b. | Thyroid storm. | f. | Iodine deficiency. |
| c. | Thyrotroph pituitary tumour. | g. | Post-thyroidectomy. |
| d. | De Quervain's thyroiditis. | h. | Drug-induced hypothyroidism. |

Match the following presentation and investigation to the most likely causative pathological process.

11) A 2-year-old boy is brought to his primary care doctor for a check-up as his family has recently emigrated from central Africa. He appears lethargic, constipated and falls below the 9th centile on growth charts. He has developed a small swelling in his neck. On further questioning, it is noted that the child was not breast fed and supplements were not given.

12) A 65-year-old Type 1 diabetic presents to her primary care doctor with a 3-month history of weight gain and leg cramps. She has noticed that her hair is dryer and she is feeling colder than before but has put this down to her age.

13) A 40-year-old female presents to her primary care doctor with episodes of dizziness and sweating. She has lost 1 stone in weight and her appetite has increased significantly. Her friends have commented that her facial features seem more prominent.

14) A 50-year-old male presents to his primary care doctor with a 2-month history of lethargy. He has put on a significant amount of weight over the past 2 months and believes his heart is beating more slowly than usual. He is concerned that this has something to do with his recent neck surgery.

15) A 20-year-old female presents with an acutely painful anterior neck swelling. She has recently had a flu-like illness which resolved 3 weeks prior to this swelling. Her pain is on the left side of her neck and is associated with fever.

## Calcium derangement

| | | | |
|---|---|---|---|
| a. | Hypocalcaemia. | e. | Tertiary hyperparathyroidism. |
| b. | Hypercalcaemia. | f. | Primary hypoparathyroidism. |
| c. | Primary hyperparathyroidism. | g. | Secondary hypoparathyroidism. |
| d. | Secondary hyperparathyroidism. | h. | Pseudo-hypoparathyroidism. |

Match the following symptoms and investigation results to the most likely disease process.

16) A 70-year-old male attends his primary care doctor for feelings of peri-oral numbness. As part of the examination he has his blood pressure measured which on inflation of the cuff on his left arm causes his left wrist to flex.

17) A patient with a background of CKD 3 and secondary hyperparathyroidism presents with a 7-day history of abdominal pain and irritability. His blood tests demonstrate a raised serum calcium, elevated PTH and raised serum phosphate.

18) A 25-year-old Asian female presents to her primary care doctor complaining of muscle spasms and occasional palpitations.

19) A 70-year-old male presents to his primary care doctor with a 6-month history of weight loss and right-sided flank pain which radiates to his groin. He is a lifelong smoker and has had a dry, non-productive cough for the past 12 months.

20) A 67-year-old male presents to his primary care doctor with muscular spasms and cramps. Routine blood tests reveal a low serum calcium and raised serum PTH.

## Adrenal disorders

| | | | |
|---|---|---|---|
| a. | Cushing's disease. | e. | Conn's syndrome. |
| b. | Ectopic ACTH secretion. | f. | Addison's disease. |
| c. | Iatrogenic steroid use. | g. | Hypoadrenalism — steroids. |
| d. | Adrenal neoplasm. | h. | Adrenocortical hyperplasia. |

Match the following patient descriptions to the most likely diagnosis.

21) A 35-year-old female presents to her primary care doctor with episodic headaches. On examination, her blood pressure is elevated at 210/150mmHg. Blood tests reveal a low serum potassium and raised serum sodium. A CT scan shows a unilateral lesion on her left adrenal gland.

22) A 65-year-old male is seen in the emergency department following a collapse. He is found to be profoundly hypotensive and complains of abdominal pain and diarrhoea for the past 24 hours. He completed a course of steroids 2 days ago.

23) A 60-year-old male presents to his primary care doctor with multiple bruises occurring on minimal trauma. He is currently under investigation for a small lung nodule. He believes his muscles have decreased in size. On examination, he has a lump at the back of his neck and multiple areas of bruising.

24) A 40-year-old female presents to her primary care doctor with darkened skin pigmentation. She notes feeling nauseous and friends have commented she appears more toned although she has not been going to the gym. On examination, she has a low blood pressure and dark lines on her palms.

25) A 35-year-old female presents to her primary care doctor with significant weight gain around her trunk. She feels her muscles are weaker than previously and feels lethargic. She is currently taking long-term steroids for early-onset rheumatoid arthritis. On examination, she has purple abdominal striae and hirsutism.

## Adrenal pathology

| | | | |
|---|---|---|---|
| a. | Phaeochromocytoma. | e. | Hypothyroidism. |
| b. | Congenital adrenal hyperplasia. | f. | Hyperthyroidism. |
| c. | Acromegaly. | g. | Type 1 diabetes mellitus. |
| d. | Hyperprolactinaemia. | h. | Type 2 diabetes mellitus. |

Match the following presentations with the most likely diagnosis.

26) A 28-year-old female presents to her primary care doctor with a difficulty conceiving for the past 2 years. She has acne and has had irregular infrequent periods for several years. Her only medical history is having some significant surgery when she was a baby but is unsure of the details.

27) A 40-year-old male presents with episodes of sweating and feeling flushed. He has frequent headaches but thought symptoms were due to stress at work. On examination, he is found to be tachycardic and hypertensive.

28) A 50-year-old male presents with a 2-month history of daily global headaches which are associated with limb pain. He has noticed a gradual change in his vision, which he describes as "tunnel vision". He mentions his rings and shoes are tighter than previously.

29) A 50-year-old lady presents with significant weight gain over the last 6 months. She feels fatigued and believes her hair is thinner than previously.

30) A 32-year-old male presents to his primary care doctor with gynaecomastia. He feels embarrassed by this condition and has noticed a difficulty in maintaining erections for the last 3 months. He has put his symptoms down to stress at work but he is concerned as he has experienced headaches and decreased libido for the past 2 weeks.

## Pituitary pathology

a.  Corticotroph tumour.                    e.  Non-functioning pituitary adenoma.
b.  Somatotroph tumour.                     f.  Pituitary infarction.
c.  Thyrotroph tumour.                      g.  Hypopituitarism — trauma.
d.  Gonadotroph tumour.                     h.  Hypopituitarism — post-irradiation.

Match the symptoms and presentation to the most likely diagnosis.

31)  A 40-year-old male presents to his primary care doctor with a loss of peripheral vision and his left eye appears to be pointing down and out. He has noted weight loss and palpitations. On examination, he has a fine tremor and tachycardia.

32)  A 25-year-old female presents to her primary care doctor 2 months post-partum. She is fatigued, pale, has dry skin and a hoarse voice. On examination, she is bradycardic and hypotensive. Routine bloods show hypoglycaemia and hyponatraemia. Her pregnancy was uneventful other than a large post-partum haemorrhage.

33)  A 50-year-old male presents with headaches which are worse on waking. He is fatigued and has developed a tingling and numbness in his right-sided little and ring finger which is worse at night and improves on shaking the hand over the edge of the bed. He also noted his skin has become rougher and his tongue appears to have increased in size.

34)  A 60-year-old male presents to his primary care doctor with muscle wasting. He noted some weight gain and has been struggling to concentrate. His past medical history includes hypertension and a traffic accident 1 year ago in which he sustained a traumatic brain injury.

35)  A 25-year-old male presents to his primary care doctor with severe headaches which are worst in the morning for the past 6 months. He notes the headache gets worse on straining to open his bowels or pass urine and on coughing. He has reported recent weight gain around his stomach and his voice has become deeper.

## Endocrine management

a.   IV hydrocortisone.
b.   Fixed-rate insulin infusion.
c.   Metformin.
d.   Gliclazide.

e.   IM glucagon 1mg.
f.   IV calcium gluconate.
g.   Alpha- and beta-blockade.
h.   Oral glucose gel.

Match the following with the most appropriate initial management.

36)   A young male attends the emergency department complaining of polyuria and polydipsia. He notes several days of abdominal pain. Blood results show hyperglycaemia and urinary ketones are positive. The attending doctor suspects a diagnosis of diabetic ketoacidosis.

37)   A 45-year-old female attends her primary care doctor complaining of thirst and multiple episodes of oral thrush. She has a BMI of 42kg/m$^2$ and does not exercise. The doctor suspects Type 2 diabetes and commences an oral medication.

38)   A 57-year-old Type 2 diabetic presents to the emergency department feeling drowsy. She has been feeling unwell for 2 days and has not been eating. She collapses in the waiting room. She is unconscious and blood glucose is 1.2mmol/L.

39)   A 40-year-old male presents with numbness and tingling around his lips. He has had severe muscle cramps and frequent spasms over the last 24 hours. Routine bloods show hypocalcaemia and magnesium within normal limits.

40)   A 70-year-old man is brought into the emergency department profoundly hypotensive. He has a known bladder tumour and has recently finished a course of reducing high-dose steroids. He has had 2L of IV fluid resuscitation with little success. The consultant caring for the patient is concerned this may be an Addisonian crisis.

## Endocrine diagnostics

| | | | | |
|---|---|---|---|---|
| a. | Type 1 diabetes. | | e. | Hypercalcaemia. |
| b. | Type 2 diabetes. | | f. | Hypocalcaemia. |
| c. | Hyperthyroidism. | | g. | Acromegaly. |
| d. | Hypothyroidism. | | h. | Addison's disease. |

Match the description of the patient with the most likely diagnosis.

41) A 45-year-old male presents to his primary care doctor with a 3-week history of fatigue, significant weight loss and reduced appetite. He looks tanned but denies any recent travel or sun exposure. He appears to have reduced muscle mass compared with previous visits. Routine bloods reveal hyponatraemia, hyperkalaemia and hypoglycaemia.

42) A 60-year-old female presents to her primary care doctor with numbness around her mouth and frequent muscle spasms. It is noted that when she has her blood pressure taken her wrist and fingers flex involuntarily.

43) A 21-year-old male presents to his primary care doctor with increased urinary frequency, excessive thirst and lethargy. His family are concerned he may be depressed but he states his mood is normal. Routine observations show an elevated serum glucose.

44) A 75-year-old male presents to the emergency department with severe abdominal pain and lethargy. He has a 2-day history of urinary frequency and dyspepsia. He appears dehydrated and has a history of lung cancer with bony metastases.

45) A 35-year-old female presents to her primary care doctor with a 3-month history of increasing fatigue, significant weight gain and cold intolerance. On examination, she has a bradycardia and has dry skin. She mentions her hair appears thinner than usual.

# Short answer questions

1) A 20-year-old male presents to the emergency department with vomiting, nausea, lethargy and abdominal pain. His blood glucose is markedly elevated and the doctor caring for the patient is concerned about diabetic ketoacidosis (DKA).

a. List two criteria that make up a diagnosis of DKA.                    1 mark
b. List two other symptoms that might be seen with DKA.                  2 marks
c. List three other signs which might be seen in DKA.                    3 marks
d. Name two other investigations for this patient.                      1 mark
e. List three initial aspects of treatment.                             3 marks

2) A 60-year-old female presents with polyuria, constipation and nausea. Bloods reveal a raised serum calcium at 3.4mmol/L.

a. Which blood tests will help to form a diagnosis?                     2 marks
b. List three other symptoms for hypercalcaemia.                       3 marks
c. What changes might be seen on an ECG of someone with severe          2 marks
   hypercalcaemia?
d. List two common causes of hypercalcaemia.                           2 marks
e. List two initial steps for hypercalcaemia management.               1 mark

3) A 70-year-old male presents to the emergency department with a 5-day history of a cough producing green sputum, fevers and rigors. He has a history of Type 2 diabetes and blood sugars are 30.2mmol/L. The consultant is concerned about a hyperosmolar hyperglycaemic state (HHS).

| | | |
|---|---|---|
| a. | What is the most likely trigger for this in this case? | 1 marks |
| b. | List three other potential symptoms of HHS. | 3 marks |
| c. | Intravenous fluid resuscitation is a key management step and is given slowly to avoid a severe complication; what is this complication? | 2 marks |
| d. | Name another important treatment in the acute phase. | 2 marks |
| e. | Name one major complication of HHS. | 2 marks |

4) A 40-year-old female presents to her primary care doctor with a neck swelling, increasing anxiety and feeling warmer than usual. Her doctor believes this patient may have hyperthyroidism.

| | | |
|---|---|---|
| a. | What is the most likely cause of the neck swelling? | 2 marks |
| b. | Name the commonest cause of this condition in the UK. | 2 marks |
| c. | List three other signs or symptoms for hyperthyroidism. | 3 marks |
| d. | List two methods of treating this condition. | 2 marks |
| e. | Name one complication of hyperthyroidism. | 1 mark |

5) A 55-year-old male presents to his primary care doctor with weight gain, fatigue and lethargy. He has a background of COPD and has recently been on a long course of prednisolone. His doctor is concerned about Cushing's syndrome.

a. What is the most likely cause of this patient's condition? 2 marks

b. Give three other signs or symptoms seen in a patient with Cushing's syndrome. 3 marks

c. Name a diagnostic test that can be used to identify Cushing's syndrome. 2 marks

d. Name one other investigation that may be considered to identify a cause of Cushing's syndrome. 2 marks

e. Name one complication of Cushing's syndrome. 1 mark

6) A 25-year-old male presents to his primary care doctor complaining of headaches. On examination, his blood pressure is 190/140mmHg. He has no medical history. His doctor is concerned about Conn's syndrome.

a. What is the pathological process behind primary Conn's syndrome? 2 marks

b. What is the most common cause of Conn's syndrome? 2 marks

c. Blood tests requested suggest Conn's syndrome. What is the next diagnostic test you would consider? 2 marks

d. Give one medical and one surgical management. 2 marks

e. List two complications of untreated Conn's syndrome. 2 marks

7) A 40-year-old female presents to her primary care doctor with fatigue and weight loss. Whilst in the waiting room she vomits and collapses. She is found to be hypotensive and tachycardic. Her doctor is concerned about an Addisonian crisis.

a. What is the main cause of primary hypoadrenalism? 1 mark
b. Give two signs that you might find in a patient with Addison's disease. 2 marks
c. What would you expect to see on blood tests for this patient's sodium, potassium and glucose? 3 marks
d. What diagnostic test would you consider to confirm a diagnosis of Addison's disease? 2 marks
e. One of the mainstays of treatment is steroids. What advice would you give about their steroid therapy? 2 marks

8) A 45-year-old male presents to his primary care doctor concerned that he is developing breast tissue. On examination, gynaecomastia is present and his doctor organises investigations to investigate a diagnosis of hyperprolactinaemia.

a. List two physiological causes of hyperprolactinaemia. 2 marks
b. List three other signs or symptoms of hyperprolactinaemia. 3 marks
c. During examination, which aspect of the cranial nerves is it important to test in hyperprolactinaemia? 2 marks
d. Which form of imaging would you consider when investigating for hyperprolactinaemia? 1 mark
e. List one medical and one surgical method for managing this. 2 marks

9)  A 50-year-old male presents to his primary care doctor as he is concerned regarding a change in his appearance. His nose is getting slowly larger and his shoes no longer fit properly. His doctor is worried he may have acromegaly.

a.  What is the most common cause of acromegaly?                                    2 marks
b.  List three other signs or symptoms found in acromegaly.                         3 marks
c.  He mentions numbness and tingling of his radial three digits of his             2 marks
    right hand. Which complication is causing this?
d.  What is the diagnostic test for acromegaly?                                     1 mark
e.  Name one medical and one surgical treatment.                                    2 marks

10) A 40-year-old female presents to the emergency department with peripheral oedema and labile hypertension. She has no medical history of note. The attending doctor is concerned about a phaeochromocytoma.

a.  Which part of the adrenal gland is affected?                                    2 marks
b.  Name one familial syndrome which includes this condition.                       2 marks
c.  Name three other signs or symptoms of this condition.                           3 marks
d.  What are the first steps in medical treatment?                                  2 marks
e.  In what proportion of people is this malignant?                                 1 marks

11) A newborn baby is referred by the midwife as she is unable to determine the sex of the baby. It is possible the child may have congenital adrenal hyperplasia (CAH).

a.  Which is the most commonly involved enzyme deficiency causing this             2 marks
    condition?
b.  List three other signs or symptoms that may be found in someone                3 marks
    with CAH.
c.  Which serum marker is raised in the most common form of this                   2 marks
    condition?
d.  Give two medical treatments for CAH.                                            2 marks
e.  What advice would you give about treatment during an acute illness?            1 mark

12) A patient presents to the emergency department severely dehydrated. You suspect they may have diabetes insipidus (DI).

|   |   |   |
|---|---|---|
| a. | Define "central" DI? | 2 marks |
| b. | Define "nephrogenic" DI. | 2 marks |
| c. | Name a drug that can cause nephrogenic DI. | 1 mark |
| d. | Would you expect raised or low values of the following in DI: sodium, plasma osmolarity, urine osmolarity? | 3 marks |
| e. | What is the diagnostic test to differentiate cranial from nephrogenic DI? | 2 marks |

13) A 75-year-old presents to his primary care doctor with a 4-month history of a dry cough and weight loss. He is now coughing up small amounts of blood, feels excessively thirsty and is passing as much urine as previously. A chest X-ray shows a small nodule in the left upper lobe. The doctor is concerned he might have the syndrome of inappropriate antidiuretic hormone (SIADH).

|   |   |   |
|---|---|---|
| a. | In this case, what is the most likely cause of SIADH? | 2 marks |
| b. | What would you expect the serum sodium to be? | 2 marks |
| c. | A urine sample is sent for analysis. What would you expect the urinary sodium and osmolarity to be — high or low? | 2 marks |
| d. | Name one method of treating this medically. | 1 mark |
| e. | Which complication can be life-threatening if the sodium level is not corrected at a controlled rate? | 3 marks |

# Chapter 6

# Neurology
## QUESTIONS

**Single best answer questions**

1) A 64-year-old female is seen in the neurology clinic as she is concerned about her memory. Her partner reports she has difficulty finding words for objects and is forgetting the names of family members. On occasion, she has forgotten conversations. You perform an Addenbrooke's Cognitive Examination in which she scores 78. MRI imaging demonstrates global atrophy. Which one of the following would not be a first-line treatment?

a. Galantamine.
b. Rivastigmine.
c. Donepezil.
d. Memantine.

2) A 73-year-old male with a history of hypertension and high cholesterol rapidly developed unilateral weakness and facial droop. He presented to the emergency department, where CT scanning confirms an acute ischaemic stroke. A 24-hour ECG monitor shows sinus rhythm and the patient has no drug allergies. Following

acute management what antiplatelet therapy would be most appropriate for the secondary prevention of stroke?

a. Dipyridamole 200mg and aspirin 75mg daily.
b. Clopidogrel 75mg daily.
c. Aspirin 75mg daily.
d. Dipyridamole 200mg daily.

3) A 21-year-old female is admitted with headache and confusion following a flu-like illness. On examination, she is disorientated, febrile and has ulcerated lesions on her lips. Her conscious level deteriorates and she develops tonic-clonic seizures. What findings are most likely?

a. Blood glucose 2.1mmol/L.
b. Lymphocytosis, normal-to-high protein, clear CSF on lumbar puncture.
c. Hyperattenuating material in the subarachnoid space on a CT of the head.
d. Raised polymorphs, high protein, low glucose and turbid cerebrospinal fluid on lumbar puncture.

4) A 79-year-old female presents to the emergency department with unilateral weakness. She tells you that she noticed the symptoms when she woke up this morning. On examination, she has marked weakness in her right arm and to a lesser degree in her right leg. She has no slurred speech or swallowing difficulties. After an initial assessment, what is the most appropriate management for this patient?

a. Urgent CT of the head and thrombolysis if an ischaemic stroke is confirmed.

b. Aspirin 300mg while awaiting a CT of the head.

c. Urgent CT of the head and aspirin 300mg within 24 hours if an ischaemic stroke is confirmed.

d. Urgent CT of the head and clopidogrel 300mg within 24 hours if an ischaemic stroke is confirmed.

5) A 24-year-old male with no previous medical history presents with dysarthria. On examination, you elicit a resting tremor. A slit-lamp examination demonstrates a brownish-yellow ring around the limbus. What biochemical results would you expect?

a. High serum ceruloplasmin and high 24-hour urinary copper.

b. Low serum ceruloplasmin and high 24-hour urinary copper.

c. Low serum ceruloplasmin and low 24-hour urinary copper.

d. High serum ceruloplasmin and low 24-hour urinary copper.

6) You are asked to see a patient with known motor neurone disease who has developed shortness of breath. He was diagnosed 18 months ago and is now fully dependent for all care. On examination, his respiratory rate is 26 and his breathing is shallow with accessory muscle use. He appears drowsy. On auscultation, the chest sounds are quiet with sounds of upper airway secretion. You perform an arterial blood gas, which shows a pH of 7.30 (7.35-7.45), a $PaO_2$ of 8.6kPa (10-14kPa), a $PaCO_2$ of 6.87kPa (4.5-6kPa), a bicarbonate of 24mmol/L (22-26mmol/L) and a lactate of 1.0mmol/L. Which of the below treatment options are most likely to be of benefit?

a. Intravenous antibiotics.

b. Salbutamol nebs.

c. Non-invasive ventilation.

d. Treatment dose low-molecular-weight heparin.

7) A 54-year-old female is admitted with loss of sensation in her right side. One year ago, she was admitted with blurred vision and pain in one eye. At that time, visual evoked potentials were delayed. Which of these is not a disease-modifying therapy used in this patient's condition?

a. Interferon beta.
b. Fingolimod.
c. Etanercept.
d. Natalizumab.

8) A 29-year-old female presents to the clinic with a several-week-long history of weakness. She feels this especially when trying to walk upstairs. She states she feels weak when washing her hair. On examination, there is no muscle wasting present and she has fatigable reflexes. What is the most likely underlying pathophysiology?

a. Degeneration of motor neurones.
b. Antibodies to acetylcholine receptor protein at the neuromuscular junction.
c. Inflammation of muscle.
d. Antibody-mediated demyelination in the central nervous system.

9) A 33-year-old female is seen in the epilepsy clinic with her partner. She has previously been diagnosed as epileptic and was started on sodium valproate. Her seizures are still happening frequently. Her partner describes them as lasting 5-10 minutes, with whole body shaking. During the clinic appointment, she slumps to the floor and has an episode lasting 4 minutes. During the episode, she makes gyrating movements and moans. Her eyes are closed

during the seizure. On coming around, she recovers quickly and is crying. She does not remember it happening. Her partner says this is typical of all her seizures. What is the most appropriate next step in her management?

a. Trial of levetiracetam.
b. Withdrawal of valproate.
c. Trial of carbamazepine.
d. Increase dose of valproate.

10) A 72-year-old female attends the clinic with her daughter who advises that she has been increasingly forgetful over several months and is slow to respond in conversation. She also reports that her mother is newly incontinent of urine. The patient's MMSE is 7/10 and she is unable to perform the 20-1 test. On examination, you note a slow, broad-based gait and brisk reflexes. Neurological examination is otherwise unremarkable. Which of the options would be the most appropriate treatment for this patient?

a. Donepezil.
b. Clopidogrel 75mg.
c. Ventriculo-peritoneal shunt.
d. Rivastigmine.

11) A 49-year-old male develops sudden-onset back pain after lifting a box of files at work. Subsequently, he develops shooting pains through the back of his thighs and into the soles of his feet. On examination, he is unable to stand on his toes and ankle reflexes are reduced. Which nerve root is most likely affected?

a.   L3.
b.   L4.
c.   L5.
d.   S1.

12) A 26-year-old female complains of a loss of pain sensation in her arms. On examination, you elicit that temperature sensation is also reduced. A spinal MRI demonstrates the presence of syringomyelia. Which spinal tracts are most likely to be affected?

a.   Spinocerebellar tract.
b.   Spinothalamic tract.
c.   Dorsal column.
d.   Corticospinal tract.

13) A 34-year-old male is woken from sleep with a severe, right-sided headache around his eye. The pain comes on over minutes and lasts around an hour. The pain is severe and makes him restless. It is associated with watering of his right eye. This is the third night in a row that this has happened. He has had this a few times before, several months ago, but had not sought help because they had gone away on their own. Which treatment below could help prevent further episodes in this patient?

a.  Verapamil.
b.  Bisoprolol.
c.  Sumatriptan.
d.  Amitriptyline.

14) A 62-year-old, left-handed male suddenly develops right-sided weakness and a difficulty in talking. On examination, power is diminished in his right arm and leg. His speech is halting and without grammar. Visual function is preserved. Which stroke syndrome would his symptoms fit best within?

a.  Total anterior circulation stroke.
b.  Partial anterior circulation stroke.
c.  Lacunar syndrome.
d.  Posterior circulation syndrome.

15) A 57-year-old female experiences spasms of severe, electric-shock-like sensations across the left side of the face. She reports that they often come on when she is cleaning her teeth and are often preceded by a feeling of numbness or tingling. You perform a neurological examination, which is normal. Which of the following medications could be used in the treatment of her headaches?

a.  Sumatriptan.
b.  Propranolol.
c.  Carbamazepine.
d.  100% oxygen.

16) A 21-year-old with focal seizures is seen in the epilepsy clinic. She is treatment-naïve and is commenced on carbamazepine as a first-line treatment for her seizures. What is the mechanism of action of carbamazepine?

a. Blocks sodium channels, inhibits gaba-transaminase, suppresses glutamate action and blocks T-type calcium channels.
b. Blocks voltage-gated sodium channels.
c. Blocks T-type calcium channels.
d. Prolongs opening of chloride channels via GABA receptors.

17) A 28-year-old female presents with weakness on a background of blurred vision and drooping eyelids. She complains of difficultly washing and brushing her hair because her arms quickly feel weak. On examination, she has a bilateral ptosis. Which of these antibodies is most likely to be positive in this patient?

a. Anti-Ro.
b. Anti-MuSK.
c. ANCA.
d. Anti-DsDNA.

18) A 47-year-old male has a 3-day history of a headache. He has been feeling progressively unwell with neck stiffness, fever and photophobia. On examination, neck stiffness and photophobia are present. You suspect meningitis and perform a lumbar puncture. Which of these would most appropriately describe the CSF findings in viral meningitis?

a.  Raised polymorphs, raised protein and low glucose.
b.  Raised lymphocytes, raised protein and low glucose.
c.  Raised polymorphs, normal protein and normal glucose.
d.  Raised lymphocytes, normal protein and normal glucose.

19) A 72-year-old female with Parkinson's disease is struggling with worsening of her symptoms before she takes her next dose of Sinemet®, which she has been taking for several years. She is prescribed selegiline to help in the management of these symptoms. What is the mechanism of action of selegiline?

a.  Inhibition of the enzyme which metabolises levodopa outside the central nervous system.
b.  Dopamine receptor agonist.
c.  Inhibition of the enzyme which metabolises dopamine.
d.  Increases dopamine release and blocks dopamine reuptake.

20) A 30-year-old known epileptic is in the emergency department following a seizure. While awaiting further assessment, you are called to see them for a further seizure. You perform an ABCDE assessment, secure their airway and give 40mg IV lorazepam. Blood glucose is normal. After 5 minutes, the patient is still seizing. What is the most appropriate next step?

a.  Give a second dose of lorazepam.
b.  Monitor for 5 more minutes, then a second dose of lorazepam.
c.  Transfer the patient to the intensive care unit.
d.  Phenytoin infusion.

21) A 31-year-old female suffers from recurrent headaches. They occur 3-4 times a month and each one lasts for several hours. She has missed multiple days off work in the last month and she is worried that she will lose her job. The headaches are one-sided and come on gradually. Before they start, she sees flashes in her vision. She was diagnosed with migraines by her primary care doctor who prescribed sumatriptan 50mg. She takes sumatriptan when she feels she is developing a headache, with minimal effect. What would be the most appropriate next step in her management?

a.   Add diclofenac suppositories.
b.   Consider investigating for an alternative cause of her headaches.
c.   Increase dose of sumatriptan.
d.   Start propranolol.

22) A 66-year-old female is seen in clinic with a several-month-long history of tremor. She describes it as worse when she is trying to use her hands. This is distressing her as tasks such as doing up buttons are difficult and she frequently spills drinks. She reports the tremor is about the same on both sides. On questioning, she thinks her father also had a similar tremor, but she can't remember what caused it. On examination, tone and power in her arms are normal and you easily elicit an intention tremor. Which of the treatments below would be most appropriate?

a.   Sinemet.
b.   Rotigotine.
c.   Propranolol.
d.   D-penicillamine.

23) A 21-year-old male is involved in a head-on road traffic collision. CT shows an intracerebral contusion. His GCS is initially 15 and he is transferred to the neurosurgery ward for monitoring. Overnight, he complains of a worsening headache and his GCS rapidly drops to 10. Pending definitive management, which of the following would not be part of the initial management?

a.  Elevate head of the bed to 30°.
b.  Aiming for a systolic blood pressure between 120-160mmHg.
c.  Mannitol.
d.  Analgesia.

# Extended matching questions

## Abnormal movement

| | | | |
|---|---|---|---|
| a. | Subthalamic stroke. | e. | Parkinson's disease. |
| b. | Huntington's disease. | f. | Simple partial seizure. |
| c. | Transient ischaemic attack. | g. | Wilson's disease. |
| d. | Benign essential tremor. | h. | Multiple sclerosis. |

Match the description of the patient with the most likely diagnosis.

1) A 67-year-old female is concerned about a tremor that she is developing in her hands. It is the same in both hands and worse when she is using her hands. She thinks her mother had a similar tremor.

2) An 82-year-old male with Type 2 diabetes and hypertension develops wild, flailing movements on one side of his body.

3) A 74-year-old male notes he is losing hand dexterity. On examination, you note a tremor in the left hand, while he performs tasks with his right hand.

4) A 79-year-old male with a history of previous strokes has two episodes of shaking in one hand, each lasting less than 2 minutes. No tremor is apparent on examination between episodes.

5) A 27-year-old female presents with a gradual onset of a tremor in both hands. Her family has also noticed that her voice has changed with variation in the speed and volume of speech.

## Visual disturbance

a.   Optic chiasm.                  e.   Left temporal lobe.
b.   Left occipital lobe.           f.   Right optic nerve.
c.   Right temporal lobe.           g.   Left parietal lobe.
d.   Left optic nerve.              h.   Right parietal lobe.

## Match the visual deficit with the site of the lesion.

6)      A right-sided homonymous inferior quadrantanopia.

7)      A left-sided central scotoma.

8)      A left-sided homonymous superior quadrantanopia.

9)      Bitemporal hemianopia.

10)     A right-sided complete visual loss.

## Headache

a.  Medication overuse.          e.  Migraine.
b.  Meningitis.                  f.  Trigeminal neuralgia.
c.  Temporal arteritis.          g.  Cluster headache.
d.  Tension headache.            h.  Space-occupying lesion.

Match the description of the patient with the most likely diagnosis.

11) A 52-year-old male has a daily headache present on waking from sleep, which eases through the day. This is associated with nausea and vomiting. It is worse on coughing.

12) A 19-year-old university student has an occipital headache, present from waking the previous morning. It is constant in nature, bilateral and radiating to the frontal region and into his neck. He describes it as a pressure sensation. He is worried as it is interfering with his revision for his upcoming exams.

13) An 18-year-old university student is brought into hospital by her flatmate with a headache. Her headache is occipital and worsens throughout the day. It radiates into her neck. She is drowsy and febrile on admission.

14) A 34-year-old female office worker has daily headaches, which feels like a tight band around her head. Occasionally the headaches are more severe and unilateral and throbbing in nature. She takes paracetamol and ibuprofen almost daily for the headaches and sumatriptan at least 4 times a week when the headaches are severe for previously diagnosed migraines with little relief.

15) A 21-year-old university student has a unilateral headache, present from waking this morning. It is severe, throbbing and worse when he sits up. He feels generally unwell, tired and photophobic. He has vomited twice.

# Weakness

| | | | |
|---|---|---|---|
| a. | Spinal metastases. | e. | Myasthenia gravis. |
| b. | Right MCA stroke. | f. | Guillain-Barré syndrome. |
| c. | Motor neurone disease. | g. | Polymyalgia rheumatica. |
| d. | Multiple sclerosis. | h. | Left MCA stroke. |

Match the description of the patient with the most likely diagnosis.

16) A 45-year-old male presents with clumsiness. He finds he tires easily when walking his dog and often trips and stumbles if he tries to run. He thinks he has lost weight recently. On examination, power is approximately 4/5 in his arms and legs. His muscles appear wasted and fasciculations are present.

17) A 72-year-old male presents with back pain and progressive bilateral leg weakness over 48 hours. Admission bloods demonstrate a raised serum corrected calcium. On examination, power is 1/5 bilaterally, reflexes are brisk and sensation is reduced.

18) A 65-year-old male presents with rapidly progressing weakness over a few days. He initially experienced some numbness and tingling in his legs before becoming unable to walk. On examination, power in the legs is markedly reduced and tendon reflexes are absent bilaterally. Power in his arms is partially reduced.

19) An 86-year-old female presents with malaise and a feeling of weakness. She has pain and stiffness in her neck, upper arms and thighs and finds it difficult to get out of bed in the morning. On examination, sensation is intact and normal power is elicited with encouragement.

20) A 39-year-old female presents with left-sided weakness and numbness. It was present from waking that morning. On examination, she has loss of power and sensation in her right leg and reduced sensation to her umbilicus. Tendon reflexes in her right leg are brisk and she has up-going plantar reflexes.

## Altered consciousness

a.  Syncope.

b.  Brain tumour.

c.  Postural hypotension.

d.  Subdural haemorrhage.

e.  Extradural haemorrhage.

f.  Epileptic seizure.

g.  Encephalitis.

h.  Non-epileptic attack.

Match the description of the patient with the most likely diagnosis.

21) A 21-year-old female becomes suddenly rigid, makes a small cry and collapses. She convulses for 1-2 minutes with symmetrical, rhythmic jerking of her limbs. She bites her tongue. There is no loss of continence. Afterwards she is drowsy and confused and cannot remember anything before being in hospital.

22) A 92-year-old female with dementia falls on the ward when getting out of a chair in an unwitnessed fall. She cannot remember what happened. There is no initial loss of consciousness and no obvious evidence of head injury on examination. Close neurological observations are commenced. When attending the patient to perform these, the nurse finds her GCS has dropped to 12.

23) A 19-year-old male presents with a headache and fever. Initially he is confused but progressively becomes drowsier.

24) A 66-year-old female lost consciousness when out shopping on a hot day with her husband. She began to feel light-headed and sweaty before losing consciousness. Her husband thinks she was unconscious for about 30 seconds. When she woke, she recovered quickly but looked pale.

25) A 25-year-old male has a recurrent loss of consciousness. His partner reports that when they happen, he slumps to the floor and makes jerking movements. This lasts for around 5 minutes. His eyes are closed and he makes moaning noises during the episodes. When the jerking has finished, he recovers quickly and cannot remember the episode.

## Stroke

| | | | |
|---|---|---|---|
| a. | Cerebral vein thrombosis. | e. | Ischaemic stroke. |
| b. | Extradural haemorrhage. | f. | Transient ischaemic attack. |
| c. | Acute subdural haemorrhage. | g. | Carotid artery dissection. |
| d. | Subarachnoid haemorrhage. | h. | Chronic subdural haemorrhage. |

Match the description of the patient with the most likely diagnosis.

26) A 52-year-old female falls when skiing and hits her head on a rock. She lost consciousness briefly, then woke up and felt well. Ten minutes later she lost consciousness again.

27) An 88-year-old female has been feeling progressively more confused over the last 2-3 weeks. When asked, she does remember falling a few weeks ago and hitting her head on the wall, but she felt fine afterwards and did not seek medical attention.

28) A 24-year-old female, who is 26 weeks' pregnant develops a sudden-onset headache, nausea and vomiting. In the emergency department, she has a seizure.

29) A 69-year-old male rapidly developed weakness in his right arm and a right facial droop. On examination in the emergency department, his pulse is irregularly irregular.

30) A 49-year-old male experiences the worst headache he has ever had. It came on over a matter of seconds and caused him to vomit. His neck is stiff.

## Cranial nerves

| | | | |
|---|---|---|---|
| a. | Cranial nerve III. | e. | Cranial nerve VII. |
| b. | Cranial nerve IV. | f. | Cranial nerve VIII. |
| c. | Cranial nerve V. | g. | Cranial nerve X. |
| d. | Cranial nerve VI. | h. | Cranial nerve XI. |

Match the description of the patient with the site of the lesion.

31) A 35-year-old female notices left facial drooping including the forehead and a loss of taste.

32) A 41-year-old female has been suffering from headaches and nausea. She has now noticed that her right eyelid is drooping. On examination, you find a right ptosis and a fixed dilated right pupil.

33) A 44-year-old male suffers from severe, electric-shock-like pain across his face lasting for a few seconds at a time.

34) A 19-year-old female hit her head after falling from a horse. She develops blurred vision when looking downwards.

35) A 59-year-old male has been having headaches that are worse in the morning for several weeks. He has now developed double vision. On examination, he cannot look outwards with his right eye.

## Seizures

a. Focal impaired awareness.
b. Non-epileptic attack.
c. Tonic-clonic seizure.
d. Focal aware seizure.

e. Akinetic seizure.
f. Absence seizure.
g. Syncope.
h. Tonic seizure.

Match the description of the patient with the most likely diagnosis.

36) A 7-year-old girl attends the clinic with her parents. They are concerned because they have noticed that she often goes vacant. Sometimes her face twitches during these episodes, which only last a few seconds. Afterwards, she carries on playing and denies that anything happened.

37) A 27-year-old male experiences episodes of jerking which start in his left hand before progressing to involve his whole arm. He is aware during the episode and feels normal afterwards.

38) A 39-year-old female has a recurrent loss of consciousness. During the episodes, she moans and slumps to the floor where she jerks rhythmically. Her eyes are closed and they last 5 minutes or more. She recovers quickly but is crying.

39) A 33-year-old male attends the clinic with his wife. She reports that he has episodes of becoming disorientated and not knowing who or where he is, before going vacant and smacking his lips for around a minute. Afterwards he cannot remember the episode but feels tired for a few minutes.

40) A 23-year-old male presents to the emergency department. His girlfriend reports that he became suddenly rigid, made a small cry and collapsed. He then made symmetrical, rhythmic jerking movements for 2-3 minutes. He had urine incontinence. In the emergency department he is drowsy and cannot remember the episode.

## Weakness

| | | | |
|---|---|---|---|
| a. | Aspirin. | e. | Methylprednisolone. |
| b. | Carbamazepine. | f. | Co-Careldopa. |
| c. | Selegiline. | g. | Pyridostigmine. |
| d. | Sumatriptan. | h. | Riluzole. |

## Match the description with the most appropriate treatment.

41) A 30-year-old female developed sudden-onset numbness and tingling, followed by weakness in her left arm and face. This lasted for 1 hour and was followed by a left-sided headache, which was severe and throbbing in nature. She felt nauseated and needed to lie down in a darkened room to wait for it to resolve.

42) A 52-year-old female has weakness that has been getting progressively worse over weeks to months. She first noticed this as a dragging of her left foot, which has caused her to trip easily. She now struggles to get up from chairs and finds stairs especially difficult. On examination, you note muscle wasting and fasciculation, most marked on the left.

43) A 72-year-old female presents to the emergency department with left-sided weakness. It came on suddenly earlier that morning. She found that she could not lift her left arm as high as the right and that the left side of her face was drooping. By the time she is seen in the emergency department, the symptoms have resolved, around 5 hours after they started.

44) A 29-year-old female presents with blurred vision that has been present for some weeks. More recently she finds that she is more generally weak, particularly towards the end of the day. In the consultation, you note a ptosis and that her words are quieter and more slurred the longer she speaks.

45) A 42-year-old female presents with right-sided leg weakness and numbness. It was present when she woke that day. This is not new to her, it being her third such episode. She has previously had right arm weakness that later resolved and prior to that an episode of blurred vision and eye pain.

## Short answer questions

1) A 62-year-old presents with a change in his gait. He is fond of painting but found this more difficult recently because he feels his dexterity is reduced. During the review, you note a resting tremor in his right hand. On examination, he has a shuffling gait, with reduced arm swing. He has difficultly performing rapid fine movements and he has increased tone and cogwheeling on the right. You suspect Parkinson's disease.

a. Describe the pathophysiology.      2 marks
b. Name one gene associated with Parkinson's disease.      1 mark
c. Give three other motor signs or symptoms you might find.      3 marks
d. Give three non-motor signs or symptoms found in this condition.      3 marks
e. Name one drug class that could be used other than levodopa.      1 mark

2) A 62-year-old heavy-goods vehicle driver attends the emergency department. Earlier in the day he noticed slurred speech and weakness in his right arm. This lasted approximately half an hour and has now completely resolved. His past medical history includes hypertension and high cholesterol. On arrival in the department his observations were as follows: saturations 98% on air, heart rate 86 bpm, blood pressure 165/92mmHg, temperature 36.7°C, respiration rate 18 breaths per

minute. You suspect he has had a transient ischaemic attack.

a. Give two further risk factors for a transient ischaemic attack.   2 marks
b. Give four tests other than bloods that may be useful.   4 marks
c. What is his ABCD2 score?   1 mark
d. What medication and dose would you give whilst awaiting specialist review?   2 marks
e. What advice regarding driving would you give the patient?   1 mark

3) A 75-year-old female presents with a 2-day history of a temporal headache. It is present all the time but worse when she brushes her hair. She has been feeling especially tired and low in mood recently. You are concerned that she may have temporal arteritis.

a. Give two further signs or symptoms that may be present.   2 marks
b. What investigation would confirm the diagnosis?   1 mark
c. Name four side effects of steroid therapy.   4 marks
d. Give two complications of temporal arteritis.   2 marks
e. She has also been complaining of stiffness and pain in her shoulders and hips. What is the most likely reason for this?   1 mark

4) A 45-year-old male presents with clumsiness and behavioural changes. He has recently had uncontrollable dancing-like movements in his hands. After genetic testing, he is diagnosed with Huntington's disease.

a.    What is the inheritance pattern of Huntington's disease?        1 mark
b.    On what chromosome is the affected gene?                        1 mark
c.    Describe the genetic mutation.                                  2 marks
d.    Give three further psychiatric symptoms that may develop.       3 marks
e.    Give three further neurological symptoms that may develop.      3 marks

5)    A 72-year-old female presents to the neurology clinic with
      memory problems. She frequently forgets the names of
      people and places and cannot remember recent
      conversations with family. This has been progressing over
      several months. She is diagnosed with Alzheimer's
      dementia.

a.    Name three other conditions which could cause these symptoms.   3 marks
b.    State the most common genetic cause of Alzheimer's disease.     1 mark
c.    Describe the pathophysiology of Alzheimer's disease.            2 marks
d.    Give two further symptoms she may be experiencing.              2 marks
e.    Name two drug classes that could help with her symptoms.        2 marks

6)    A 69-year-old male presents with weakness. He first
      noticed that it was difficult to use his keys and now finds
      that he frequently drops or cannot grasp objects. He is
      being investigated for motor neurone disease (MND).

a.    Name two genes associated with motor neurone disease.              2 marks
b.    State three other findings for lower motor neurone involvement.    3 marks
c.    Give three other findings for upper motor neurone involvement.     3 marks
d.    Name a non-pharmacological intervention that can increase life-    1 mark
      expectancy.
e.    Name the only drug that affects life expectancy in MND.            1 mark

7) A 65-year-old male is admitted with paraplegia and back pain. He has been getting back pain for several weeks, which has been constant and wakes him from sleep. Over the past week he has had recurrent falls. This morning, he could not move his legs to get out of bed.

a.   Give two potential causes for spinal cord compression.      2 marks
b.   What investigation should help diagnose the condition?      1 mark
c.   Give one definitive treatment.                             1 mark
d.   Give three further treatments for symptom relief.          3 marks
e.   Name three possible complications that may occur.          3 marks

8) A 78-year-old female presents with paralysis and sensory loss in her right face and arm as well as dysphasia. Her husband called for an ambulance instantly. When she is seen in the emergency department her symptoms have been present for 30 minutes.

a.   Which artery is most likely occluded?                      1 mark
b.   Within what time-frame is thrombolysis considered?         1 mark
c.   Name four contraindications to thrombolysis.               4 marks
d.   What medication should be given urgently once haemorrhagic stroke   1 mark
     is excluded, if the patient is not a suitable candidate for thrombolysis?
e.   Give three drug classes used in the secondary prevention of stroke   3 marks
     following an acute stroke or TIA.

9) A 20-year-old female is brought into the emergency department after having a seizure in the supermarket. Her girlfriend was with her at the time and reports she made a cry, collapsed and went rigid before shaking rhythmically for a couple of minutes. It has never happened before, and she is not taking any regular medications. In the emergency department, she is drowsy and confused. You suspect a generalised tonic-clonic seizure.

a. Name four appropriate blood tests to perform.     4 marks

b. When she is ready to leave, she asks if it is safe for her to drive home.  2 marks
What advice regarding driving should you give her?

c. As a child, her parents told her she sometimes had "vacant episodes"  1 mark
where she would stare blankly for up to 30 seconds. She would then
resume normal activity. What is this type of seizure?

d. Name the investigation you would have performed for her at the time  2 marks
and the finding you would expect.

e. Name one appropriate first-line medication to manage the seizure  1 mark
disorder she had as a child.

10) A 32-year-old female presents with blurred vision and drooping eyelids. On examination, she has a bilateral ptosis and is unable to keep her eyes looking up during the H test for more than a few seconds. You suspect myasthenia gravis.

a. Give four further clinical features that may be seen in a patient with  4 marks
myasthenia gravis.

b. Name two antibodies which may be positive.     2 marks

c. Name one further investigation which would aid in diagnosis.     1 mark

d. Name two pharmacological treatment options.     2 marks

e. Name one non-pharmacological treatment option.     1 mark

11) A 45-year-old male presents to the emergency department with a sudden-onset, severe, occipital headache. He describes it as like being hit around the back of the head with a hammer. He has had several headaches over the last week, but each has gone away after a few minutes. An urgent CT demonstrates a subarachnoid haemorrhage.

a.   What is the most likely underlying cause of the bleed?                          1 mark
b.   If a CT scan did not detect a subarachnoid haemorrhage, what   2 marks
     investigation should be performed and what would you expect to
     find?
c.   What two investigations could locate the origin of the bleed?        2 marks
d.   What is the most likely cause of the headaches he was getting prior to   1 mark
     the one that brought him to hospital?
e.   Give two potential sequelae and the management of each.              4 marks

12) An 18-year-old student is brought into the emergency department by her flatmates. She has been complaining of a headache and fever. On examination, she is drowsy with neck stiffness and photophobia. Her temperature is 38.4°C. You suspect she may have meningitis.

a.   Why would you perform a CT of the head before doing a lumbar   1 mark
     puncture?
b.   Give three expected features in the CSF for bacterial meningitis.   3 marks
c.   Name two of the most common causative organisms for bacterial   2 marks
     meningitis in adults.
d.   What would be your immediate management for this patient in the   1 mark
     emergency department?
e.   Name two short-term complications and one long-term complication   3 marks
     that may arise from meningitis.

13) A 47-year-old female presents with a daily headache and blurred vision worsening over several months. You are concerned that she may have a space-occupying lesion.

a. Name two features of the headache that would be suggestive of a space-occupying lesion.     2 marks

b. On examination, she cannot look laterally with her left eye. What structure has likely been affected?     1 mark

c. Name four further clinical features that may be associated with a brain tumour.     4 marks

d. What investigation would you request?     1 mark

e. Name two treatment options for a primary brain tumour.     2 marks

# Chapter 7

# Haematology
## QUESTIONS

## Single best answer questions

1) Which chromosomal translocation is described as the Philadelphia chromosome, found in chronic myeloid leukaemia (CML) which encodes for a tyrosine kinase?

a. t(9:22).
b. t(11:14).
c. t(8:14).
d. t(15:17).

2) A primary care doctor reviews tests for a 60-year-old male reporting vague symptoms. The results are found below. What is the likely diagnosis?

Hb 144g/L
Neutrophils 4.3 x 10⁹/L
Sodium 136mmol/L
Urea 4.5mmol/L
Adjusted calcium 2.35mmol/L

Platelets 324 x 10⁹/L
WCC 7.2 x 10⁹/L
Potassium 4.5mmol/L
Creatinine 67µmol/L
M protein detected 15mg/L

Bone marrow aspirate: no pathological changes.

a.   Myeloma.
b.   Solitary plasmacytoma.
c.   Acute myeloid leukaemia.
d.   Monoclonal gammopathy of unknown significance (MGUS).

3)   A Thai female with hereditary spherocytosis attends her primary care doctor with a rash on her face, tiredness and breathlessness. Her blood tests can be seen below. What organism is she likely to be infected with?

Hb 45g/L                          Neutrophils 0.7 x $10^9$/L
Platelets 40 x $10^9$/L          WCC 1.3 x $10^9$/L
MCV 62fL

a.   *P. falciparum.*
b.   Influenza A.
c.   *Streptococcus viridians.*
d.   Parvovirus B19.

4)   A blood film taken from an elderly male shows teardrop poikilocytes. He has complained of fatigue and weight loss over the past few months. His haemoglobin is 89g/L. What is the likely diagnosis?

a.   Anaemia of chronic disease.
b.   Chronic lymphoblastic leukaemia.
c.   Myelofibrosis.
d.   Alcohol excess.

5) A 62-year-old male attends his primary care doctor with exertional breathlessness and chest pain. Screening blood tests are sent which show a Hb of 72g/L, MCV 65fL, $B_{12}$ and folate are normal, serum ferritin levels are 10μg/L. You suspect iron deficiency anaemia. What treatment is indicated?

a. 1 unit red cell transfusion.
b. Ferrous sulphate 200mg tds.
c. Iron infusion.
d. 1 unit red cell transfusion followed by commencement of ferrous sulphate.

6) Low-molecular-weight heparin (LMWH) can be used for prophylaxis of venous thromboembolism. What is the action of LMWH?

a. Vitamin K antagonist.
b. Factor X inhibitor.
c. Thrombin inhibitor.
d. Anti-thrombin and anti-Xa.

7) Warfarin is a vitamin K antagonist. Which clotting factors does it not inhibit the production of?

a. Factor II.
b. Factor XI.
c. Factor IX.
d. Factor X.

8) Bleeding from gums and easy bruising is typical of which condition?

a. Haemophilia A.
b. Haemophilia B.
c. Disseminated intravascular coagulation.
d. von Willebrand's disease.

9) An 8-year-old male presents to the emergency department with a painful and swollen knee, after falling on it playing in the garden. His brother had a similar presentation when he was five. Following further investigations, you diagnose the child with haemophilia A. What is the appropriate long-term treatment for this condition?

a) Recombinant factor VIII replacement.
b) Recombinant factor IX replacement.
c) Regular platelet transfusions.
d) Regular cryoprecipitate infusions.

10) A 55-year-old female presents to her primary care doctor for the results of her recent blood tests. She has no change in bowel habit or diet. She has a past medical history of Graves' disease. Routine blood results are shown below. What is the most likely diagnosis?

| | |
|---|---|
| Hb 90g/L | MCV 108fL |
| Platelets 340 x $10^9$/L | Folate 4µg/L |
| Neutrophils 3.5 x $10^9$/L | $B_{12}$ 100ng/L |
| WCC 4.5 x $10^9$/L | Ferritin 86µg/L |

a. Coeliac disease.
b. Pernicious anaemia.
c. $B_{12}$ deficiency.
d. Whipple's disease.

11) What is the most common thrombophilia in the general population?

a.   Factor V Leiden.
b.   Protein C deficiency.
c.   Protein S deficiency.
d.   Anti-thrombin III deficiency.

12) A patient presents with a painful and swollen left calf. She also complains of a pleuritic sounding chest pain. ECG shows sinus tachycardia. She is pregnant. Which investigation should be done first?

a.   V/Q scan.
b.   CT pulmonary angiogram.
c.   USS Doppler left leg.
d.   D-dimer.

13) A patient presents to the emergency department for assessment having vomited blood She has noticed easily bruising and a purpuric rash for some time. Bloods results are shown below. You think that she may have idiopathic thrombocytopenic purpura (ITP). The patient is haemodynamically stable. You do not think the bleed is life-threatening. What would be the appropriate management?

Hb 115g/L                     Platelets 14 x 10$^9$/L
Neutrophils 3.7 x 10$^9$/L     WCC 4.3 x 10$^9$/L

a.   Platelet transfusion.
b.   Ask advice from a haematologist.
c.   Start corticosteroids.
d.   Arrange a splenectomy.

14) Which of the below are not present in multiple myeloma?

a. Lytic bone lesions.
b. Renal impairment.
c. Anaemia.
d. Heavy chains in urine.

15) Which of the below conditions is not a cause of an eosinophilia?

a. Ascariasis (round worm).
b. Eczema.
c. Sarcoidosis.
d. Amyloidosis.

16) The intrinsic pathway is best monitored by measurement of which of the following?

a. PT.
b. APTT.
c. INR.
d. Fibrinogen.

17) What specific type of lymphoma is associated with the human immunodeficiency virus?

a. Burkitt's lymphoma.
b. Primary effusion lymphoma.
c. Hodgkin's lymphoma.
d. Plasmablastic lymphoma.

18) Tumour lysis syndrome is most frequently seen when high-volume chemo-sensitive disease is treated. If someone is at high risk of tumour lysis syndrome what treatment should be given prophylactically?

a.  No treatment.
b.  Rasburicase.
c.  Uric acid.
d.  Calcium.

19) Which of the below conditions is not known to cause splenomegaly?

a.  Glandular fever.
b.  Portal hypertension.
c.  Myelofibrosis.
d.  Iron deficiency anaemia.

20) Which of the following should be used as a prophylactic antibiotic in a patient who has had a splenectomy and with no drug allergies?

a.  Penicillin V.
b.  Trimethoprim.
c.  Flucloxacillin.
d.  Co-amoxiclav.

21) Which of these haematological features are not seen in microangiopathic haemolytic anaemia?

a.  Anaemia.
b.  Helmet cells.
c.  Leucocytosis.
d.  Reticulocytes.

22) Which of the below is not associated with a macrocytosis?

a.   Excess alcohol ingestion.
b.   Methotrexate.
c.   Pregnancy.
d.   Ferrous sulphate.

23) Which of the below are not blood groups?

a.   ABO.
b.   Kell.
c.   Duffy.
d.   Croft.

# Extended matching questions

## Blood films/stains

a.  Teardrop poikilocytes.
b.  Helmet cells.
c.  Heinz bodies.
d.  Ring sideroblasts.

e.  Pencil cells.
f.  Spherocytes.
g.  Prickle cells.
h.  Smear cells.

Match the description of the disease with the most likely finding on examination of a blood film.

1)  A 55-year-old male with a poor diet; he eats very little spinach or red meat. Blood tests show a microcytic anaemia.

2)  A Mediterranean teenager who had significant neonatal jaundice is thought to have haemolysed due to ingestion of fava beans.

3)  An elderly male who has frequent infections and painless lymphadenopathy. The WCC is very high.

4)  Fibrin strands are deposited in vessels; this results in damage to red cells. This disease is known as microangiopathic haemolytic anaemia.

5)  An elderly female with pancytopenia, fatigue, weight loss and sweats. On examination, there is splenomegaly.

## Risk factors for haematological conditions

| | | | |
|---|---|---|---|
| a. | Down's syndrome. | e. | MGUS. |
| b. | Polycythaemia rubra vera (PRV). | f. | SLE. |
| c. | Immunosuppression. | g. | Family history. |
| d. | Eczema. | h. | HRT. |

## Which risk factor is most associated with each condition?

6)      Acute lymphoblastic leukaemia.

7)      Chronic myeloid leukaemia.

8)      Idiopathic thrombocytopenic purpura.

9)      Non-Hodgkin's lymphoma.

10)     Haemophilia.

## Ann Arbor staging of Hodgkin's lymphoma.

a.  Stage 1.                 e.  Stage 1B.
b.  Stage 2.                 f.  Stage 2B.
c.  Stage 3.                 g.  Stage 3B.
d.  Stage 4.                 h.  Stage 4B.

## Stage the lymphoma described.

11) Lymphoma present in coeliac and mediastinal lymph nodes, asymptomatic.

12) Lymphoma isolated to the anterior cervical chain, with >10% weight loss over a period of 6 months.

13) Lymphoma present in the external/internal iliac lymph nodes, coeliac plexus and mediastinal lymph nodes. There are also deposits in the liver. The patient has night sweats and extensive weight loss.

14) A single axillary lymph node, no spread and otherwise asymptomatic.

15) A 56-year-old patient presents with a perforated appendix. Histology shows lymphoma present in the tissue of the appendix. Staging scans show this is an isolated finding. The patient has no fever, weight loss or night sweats.

## Clotting pathways

a. Factor III.
b. Factor V.
c. Factor VIII.
d. Factor IX.

e. Factor Xa.
f. Factor XII.
g. Factor XIII.
h. Anti-thrombin.

## Match the component of the clotting pathway which best fills the gap.

16) Tissue damage exposes collagen. _____ binds exposed collagen, activating the intrinsic pathway.

17) _____ is deficient in Christmas disease.

18) Apixaban and rivaroxaban are inhibitors of _____.

19) Tissue factor is otherwise known as _____. This binds factor 7 to activate the extrinsic pathway.

20) Thrombin converts fibrinogen to fibrin. Polymers of fibrin form fibrin cross links. _____ stabilises the fibrin clot.

## Abnormal clotting screens

a.  DIC.
b.  Heparin.
c.  Deficient factor II.
d.  von Willebrand's disease.

e.  Aspirin.
f.  Warfarin.
g.  Pulmonary embolism.
h.  Ticagrelor.

Match the results of the clotting screen with the likely cause.

21) Elevated APTT only.

22) Elevated PT only.

23) Elevated PT and APTT only.

24) Elevated PT, APTT, low fibrinogen and thrombocytopenia.

25) Normal clotting screen, but easy bruising and bleeding gums.

## Inherited conditions

a.   Alpha thalassaemia major.         e.   G6PD deficiency.
b.   Beta thalassaemia major.          f.   Pyruvate kinase deficiency.
c.   Haemophilia A.                    g.   Factor V Leiden.
d.   Sickle cell disease.              h.   Factor C deficiency.

## Match the statement with the most likely diagnosis.

26) Results in hydrops fetalis, which is incompatible with life.

27) A point adenine for thymine substitution, results in the amino acid glutamic acid being substituted for valine. Valine is hydrophobic.

28) The most common cause of venous thromboembolism in the general population.

29) X-linked disorder resulting in neonatal jaundice, more common in Mediterranean individuals.

30) Treatment is with regular blood transfusions and desferrioxamine.

## Abnormal blood films/stains 2

a.  Howell-Jolly bodies.          e.  Fragmented cells.
b.  Basophilic stippling.          f.  Pencil cells.
c.  Auer rods.                     g.  Teardrop cells.
d.  Sickle cells.                  h.  Heinz bodies.

Match the below with the most likely finding on a blood film.

31) Beta thalassaemia.

32) Sickle cell anaemia.

33) Post-splenectomy.

34) Mechanical heart valves.

35) Myelofibrosis.

## Blood cells

| | | | |
|---|---|---|---|
| a. | Neutrophils. | e. | Reticulocytes. |
| b. | T-helper cells. | f. | Megakaryocytes. |
| c. | B cells. | g. | Pro-normoblasts. |
| d. | Cytotoxic T cells. | h. | Eosinophils. |

Match the description of the appearance and function with the appropriate blood cell.

36) Has the marker CD4+ on its cell surface.

37) Has distinctive nuclei with up to five lobes, a few mitochondria and significant glycogen stores.

38) Bilobed nucleus, produces histamine.

39) The precursor to this cell is called a normoblast.

40) Thousands of platelets can be produced from one of these cells.

## Haemolytic anaemia

a.   Hereditary spherocytosis.

b.   Hereditary elliptocytosis.

c.   G6PD deficiency.

d.   Pyruvate kinase deficiency.

e.   Mechanical heart valve.

f.   ABO incompatibility.

g.   March haemoglobinuria.

h.   Warm autoimmune haemolytic anaemia.

Match the description of the patient with the most likely cause of haemolysis.

41)   A 47-year-old female with SLE is found to have a Hb of 47g/L. She also notes her skin has become more yellow.

42)   A 32-year-old male does an ultra marathon. His urine changed colour.

43)   Abnormal glycolytic pathway in which there is a lack of ATP production. Red cells are rigid and destroyed. Poikilocytosis and prickle cells can be seen on blood film examination.

44)   A Mediterranean male presents with a change in urine colour and a haemoglobin of 53g/L. He describes recently having severe pneumonia.

45)   Spectrin, a cytoskeletal protein, is defective. The red cells become less deformable and haemolysis occurs.

## Short answer questions

1) A 67-year-old male presents with back pain and new bilateral leg weakness to the emergency department. MRI shows malignant spinal cord compression with multiple lytic lesions in the spine. It is thought that the most likely diagnosis is multiple myeloma.

   a. Specify three other investigations to help confirm a diagnosis of myeloma.    3 marks

   b. What is a Bence Jones protein?    1 mark

   c. Describe the pathological process resulting in myeloma.    2 marks

   d. Which condition causes a paraproteinaemia with no evidence of myeloma?    2 marks

   e. What treatment is given to patients with myeloma to treat their disease and what is offered for bone protection purposes?    2 marks

2) A 65-year-old female is noted to have a high WCC and is anaemic. She has had non-specific symptoms of sweating, tiredness and weight loss. Blood tests are performed which can be seen below. Karyotyping of white cells shows the Philadelphia chromosome is present.

   Hb 95g/L
   Platelets 100 x $10^9$/L
   WCC 245 x $10^9$/L

a. What is the most likely diagnosis? 1 mark
b. What translocation causes the Philadelphia chromosome? 2 marks
c. What abnormal gene does the Philadelphia chromosome code for? 1 mark
d. What drug has revolutionised the treatment of this condition? 4 marks
   Describe the pharmacology of this drug.
e. What other condition can this disease transform to and is the 2 marks
   prognosis better or worse?

3) A 72-year-old male is discharged from hospital after having had an ischaemic stroke. He has AF and is started on warfarin to reduce the risk of further strokes. After commencement he has a stable INR.

a. Describe four criteria used in the HAS-BLED score. 4 marks
b. What would be the target INR for this patient? 1 mark

The same patient presents to the emergency department with a history of melaena, his Hb is 105g/L, urea is 20.4mmol/L, creatinine is 85μmol/L, and INR is 4.5.

c. If there is no evidence of bleeding, but the patient is at a high risk of 1 mark
   bleeding, what treatment should be given?
d. If there is a massive haemorrhage what is the treatment? 1 mark
e. What three antibiotics may have been started? 3 marks

4) An 18-year-old boy presents to primary care with a painless lump in his neck. This has been present for over 2 months now. A diagnosis of Hodgkin's lymphoma is made following further investigations.

| | | |
|---|---|---|
| a. | How would the diagnosis of lymphoma be made? | 1 mark |
| b. | What is the name of the staging system for lymphoma? | 1 mark |
| c. | Name the three B symptoms of lymphoma and two other symptoms that may be described by the patient. | 5 marks |
| d. | Histology shows a giant cell with twin mirror image uncle and prominent owl's eye nucleoli. What is the name of this formation? | 1 mark |
| e. | What blood test may be raised in Hodgkin's lymphoma? | 2 marks |

5) A 1-year-old boy from Ghana presents to the emergency department screaming. He is thought to be having a pain crisis related to sickle cell anaemia.

| | | |
|---|---|---|
| a. | Describe the inheritance of sickle cell anaemia. | 1 mark |
| b. | Describe how sickle cell anaemia causes damage to tissues and give two examples of common precipitants. | 3 marks |
| c. | Name two acute complications of sickle cell anaemia. | 2 marks |
| d. | Why does sickle cell anaemia often present in >1-year-old children? | 2 marks |
| e. | What causes a pain crisis and how is it treated? | 2 marks |

6) A 62-year-old female is admitted to hospital due to the development of a pulmonary embolism. She is tachycardic and requires 35% oxygen to maintain her saturations. She is commenced on LMWH before discharge. You see her in the anticoagulation clinic.

a. Name four symptoms that she may have complained of. 2 marks

b. What two scoring systems are used to stratify the risk of PE and what 3 marks blood test can be used alongside this?

c. What is the most frequent ECG change seen in PE? 1 mark

d. Name four tests to investigate unprovoked VTE. 2 marks

e. It is proven to be an unprovoked PE; how long should this patient 2 marks remain on anticoagulation?

7) A 32-year-old female is admitted to the emergency department with a massive delayed postpartum haemorrhage. On arrival her HR is 140 bpm and her blood pressure is 75/42mmHg. She is drowsy. Her blood group is unknown.

a. Describe your initial assessment. 2 marks

b. What type of blood (ABO) should you give this lady in the emergency 2 marks setting?

c. You find out her blood group is A-. Which group (ABO) could be given? 2 marks

d. Describe two potential complications of blood transfusion. 2 marks

e. Describe the constituents of fresh frozen plasma and cryoprecipitate. 2 marks

8) A patient on the ward becomes unwell. She is pyrexial, tachycardic and hypotensive. She notes a new productive cough, and now has an oxygen requirement. The junior doctor believes she has disseminated intravascular coagulation (DIC). This is a very dangerous condition in which the patient is both prone to bleeding and thromboses.

a. Describe the pathophysiology of DIC, explaining why the patient is 3 marks both hypercoagulable and hypocoagulable.

b. What is typically seen on blood tests in DIC? 1 mark

c. Name two triggers of DIC. 2 marks

d. Why is D-dimer raised on these blood tests? 2 marks

e. What may be seen on a blood film in DIC? 2 marks

9) A Mediterranean boy is seen by paediatricians to investigate his persistent anaemia. On examination, he is noted to have frontal bossing. He is found to have beta thalassaemia.

a. Describe the abnormality resulting in beta thalassaemia. Genetically, 2 marks what is the difference between beta thalassaemia major and the beta thalassaemia trait?

b. What may be seen on a blood film in beta thalassaemia? 3 marks

c. How might beta thalassaemia be treated? 1 mark

d. Describe four symptoms of iron overload. 2 marks

e. What treatment can be given to prevent iron overload? 2 marks

10) A 24-year-old male is given a stem cell transplant for potentially curative treatment of acute lymphoblastic leukaemia.

a. What is the difference between allogenic and autogenic stem cell 2 marks transplants?

b. What two management considerations should take place when a 2 marks patient receives a stem cell transplant?

c. Name four complications of an allogenic stem cell transplant. 2 marks

d. What is graft versus host disease? Name two organs which can be 3 marks affected.

e. What type of hypersensitivity is graft versus host disease? 1 mark

11) A mother brings her daughter to her primary care doctor because she has noted persistent easy bruising, a non-blanching rash and bleeding from the gums. You think she might have von Willebrand's disease.

a.  What is von Willebrand's factor, and what role does von Willebrand's    3 marks
    factor have in clotting?
b.  How is von Willebrand's disease inherited?    1 mark
c.  What is the abnormality in von Willebrand's disease?    2 marks

A few weeks later, a 2-year-old boy presents to the same practitioner with an acutely swollen knee. Examination is consistent with a haemarthrosis. His father had died after a significant postoperative bleed, but his mother is well.

d.  What is the likely diagnosis?    2 marks
e.  How is this disease inherited?    2 marks

12) A 72-year-old female has her annual blood tests, which are shown below.

Hb 188g/L                          Platelets 534 x 10$^9$/L
WCC 14.6 x 10$^9$/L                MCV 75.0fL
Haematocrit 68%

a.  What is the most likely diagnosis?    2 marks
b.  What genetic defect most commonly causes this disease?    2 marks
c.  Name two causes of secondary polycythaemia.    2 marks
d.  How might this condition be managed?    1 mark
e.  Name two complications of this condition and which malignant    3 marks
    disease is the patient at risk of in the future?

13) You are asked to review a 42-year-old female who is day 4 post-allogenic stem cell transplant for treatment of CML. She is pyrexial, tachycardic and tachypnoeic. Her blood pressure is 103/54mmHg. She is coughing profusely and has a new oxygen requirement with saturations 94% on 10L via a Hudson mask. Her blood results are shown below.

Hb 78g/L     Platelets 26 x $10^9$/L

WCC 0.2 x $10^9$/L   Neutrophils 0.2 x $10^9$/L

a. What would your initial assessment be?     1 mark

b. Describe four other investigations you should do.  2 marks

c. What treatment would you give her immediately?  2 marks

d. What groups of infection would you consider in light of her significant 3 marks immunosuppression?

e. A high-resolution CT shows bilateral ground glass changes. What is 2 marks the most likely diagnosis?

# Chapter 8

# Rheumatology
## QUESTIONS

## Single best answer questions

1) A 57-year-old female with a history of haemochromatosis develops sudden-onset swelling and tenderness over the base of her right thumb. A diagnosis of pseudogout is suspected. What is the composition of the crystals seen in this disease?

a. Calcium oxalate.
b. Monosodium urate.
c. Calcium pyrophosphate.
d. Struvite.

2) Which of the following HLA types is associated with rheumatoid arthritis?

a. HLA B27.
b. HLA DR4.
c. HLA DR5.
d. HLA D52.

3) A 27-year-old male of Turkish descent presents to his primary care doctor with painful genital ulcers of a 1-week duration. On further questioning he reports recurrent mouth ulcers. A diagnosis of Behçet's syndrome is made. Which of the following symptoms is he most likely to experience?

a. Eye pain.
b. Fever.
c. Erectile dysfunction.
d. Lymphadenopathy.

4) A 70-year-old female is diagnosed with giant cell arteritis. Which of the following conditions is she more at risk of developing?

a. Polymyalgia rheumatica.
b. Sjögren syndrome.
c. Dermatomyositis.
d. SLE.

5) Which of the following is associated with neonatal heart block?

a. Anti-Jo-1 and Anti-La.
b. Anti-Sm.
c. Anti-dsDNA and Anti-Ro.
d. Anti-Ro and Anti-La.

6) In rheumatoid arthritis, which of these is associated with a worse prognosis?

a. Male.
b. Smoking.
c. Acute onset.
d. HLA-B27.

7) Which of the following patients should be started on allopurinol?

a. A 72-year-old male with gout. He has had an attack of gout once 5 years ago but is otherwise fit and well with no past medical history.
b. A 65-year-old female with her first attack of gout and CKD3.
c. A 74-year-old male with high serum urate levels.
d. A 55-year-old obese male with his first presentation of gout.

8) Which of the following describes Felty's syndrome?

a. Rheumatoid arthritis, pulmonary fibrosis and eosinophilia.
b. Fevers, joint pain and salmon-coloured rash.
c. Rheumatoid arthritis, splenomegaly and neutropenia.
d. Joint pains, purpuric rash and glomerulonephritis.

9) Which of the following disease-modifying anti-rheumatic drugs (DMARDs) is most likely to cause retinopathy?

a. Leflunomide.
b. Sulfasalazine.
c. Methotrexate.
d. Hydroxychloroquine.

10) Which of the following is not associated with ankylosing spondylitis?

a.  Urethritis.
b.  Uveitis.
c.  Aortitis.
d.  Enthesitis.

11) What drug should be given to patients with giant cell arteritis (to reduce the risk of stroke)?

a.  Aspirin.
b.  Warfarin.
c.  Rivaroxaban.
d.  Low-molecular-weight heparin.

12) What is the name given to the syndrome of massive lung fibrosis in patients with rheumatoid arthritis and pneumoconiosis?

a.  Reiter's syndrome.
b.  Still's disease.
c.  Caplan syndrome.
d.  Bruns syndrome.

13) Which of the following infective agents is least associated with reactive arthritis?

a.  *Campylobacter jejuni.*
b.  *Salmonella spp.*
c.  *Chlamydia trachomatis.*
d.  *Trichomoniasis vaginalis.*

14) What is the mechanism of action of allopurinol?

a. Xanthine oxidase inhibitor.
b. Xanthine oxidase agonist.
c. Increased renal urate excretion.
d. Recombinant uricase.

15) A 76-year-old female undergoes a DEXA scan which reveals osteoporosis. What is her T-score?

a. $\leq$-2.5.
b. $\leq$-1.
c. $\geq$1.
d. $\geq$2.5.

16) A 45-year-old male presents with testicular pain and myalgia. He reveals he has lost 5kg in the last month and feels feverish. On examination, you note a mottled reticulated purple discolouration of the legs and hypertension. What is the most likely diagnosis?

a. SLE.
b. Polyarteritis nodosum.
c. Wegener's granulomatosis.
d. Henoch-Schönlein purpura.

17) What is the most common viral infection associated with polyarteritis nodosum?

a. Epstein-Barr virus.
b. HIV.
c. Hepatitis B virus.
d. Hepatitis C virus.

18) A 76-year-old female is diagnosed with giant cell arteritis and is started on prednisolone. What is the most appropriate treatment to reduce the risk of osteoporotic fractures?

a.   Lifestyle advice.
b.   Strontium ranelate.
c.   Vitamin D and calcium supplementation.
d.   Alendronate.

19) A 32-year-old male with ankylosing spondylitis complains of increasing lower back pain. He takes naproxen and is compliant with physiotherapy. What drug should now be offered?

a.   TNF-alpha inhibitors.
b.   Long-term steroids.
c.   Methotrexate.
d.   No treatment has proven benefit.

20) A 76-year-old male presents to his primary care doctor with a right-sided temporal headache which is tender to palpation. What investigation would most support a diagnosis of giant cell arteritis?

a.   Normocytic anaemia.
b.   Elevated CRP.
c.   Elevated ESR.
d.   Elevated alkaline phosphatase.

21) A 34-year-old female with SLE presents with recurrent miscarriages. A diagnosis of secondary antiphospholipid syndrome is suspected. Which of the following autoantibodies is not part of the laboratory criteria for diagnosing antiphospholipid syndrome?

a. Lupus anticoagulant.
b. Anti-cardiolipin antibody.
c. Anti-beta-2 glycoprotein 1 antibodies.
d. Anti-topoisomerase antibodies.

22) A 44-year-old female complains of pain and stiffness in her left wrist, left 3rd PIP joint and 3rd and 4th right PIP joints. A diagnosis of psoriatic arthritis is suspected. Which of the following patterns of joint involvement describes her presentation?

a. Arthritis mutilans.
b. Oligoarticular.
c. Polyarticular.
d. Spondyloarthropathy.

23) A 17-year-old boy is brought to the clinic by his mother as she is concerned he doesn't "look right". He is 186cm tall with a slim build. He has long arms and fingers and when you ask him to make a fist, his thumb extends beyond the ulnar border. Out of the following options, what is the most likely diagnosis?

a. Ehlers-Danlos syndrome.
b. Fragile X syndrome.
c. Klinefelter syndrome.
d. Marfan syndrome.

# Extended matching questions

## Connective tissue disorders

a.  SLE.
b.  Drug-induced lupus.
c.  Dermatomyositis.
d.  Polymyositis.

e.  Limited scleroderma.
f.  Sjögren syndrome.
g.  Diffuse scleroderma.
h.  Raynaud's phenomenon.

Match the description of the patient with the most likely diagnosis.

1)  A 69-year-old female with a history of hypothyroidism develops weakness, worse when walking up the stairs and brushing her hair. She is noted to have scaly papules over her knuckles.

2)  A 54-year-old male with a history of gastric reflux presents with intermittent painful white fingers. This usually occurs after working outside in the garden and he says his fingers become red when he comes inside. On examination, you note multiple dilated capillaries on his cheeks.

3)  A 60-year-old female presents with a rash on her cheeks and nose, and pain in her knees. She has recently been diagnosed with TB and is undergoing treatment. Her mother had rheumatoid arthritis and she is worried her symptoms may be due to that.

4)  A 53-year-old female presents to her primary care doctor with vaginal dryness. On further questioning, she reports a difficulty wearing her contact lenses and problems swallowing food.

5)  A 54-year-old female has a 4-month history of increasing fatigue. She has noticed an itchy, red rash on her face and generalised muscle and joint aches. She has a background of hypertension and has recently been started on amlodipine.

## Patterns of joint involvement

a.  Prepatellar bursitis.

b.  Ankylosing spondylitis.

c.  Rheumatoid arthritis.

d.  Reactive arthritis.

e.  Osteoarthritis.

f.  Osgood-Schlatter disease.

g.  Psoriatic arthritis.

h.  Gout.

## Match the description of the patient with the most likely diagnosis.

6)  A 76-year-old male presents with an insidious onset of DIP joint pain. He is writing a novel and notices the pain is worse after a long session of typing. He has no other symptoms or past medical history of note.

7)  A 47-year-old male presents with an acute onset of right knee pain. He cannot think of any precipitating factors for the pain and has a sedentary lifestyle, working in an office with no exercise.

8)  A 27-year-old female complains of morning stiffness and pain in the joints of her hands. On examination, you note DIP joint swelling in both hands.

9)  A 23-year-old male presents with insidious onset pain in his left knee. The pain is worse in the morning and improves with activity. The only past medical history of note is a recent cold.

10) A 30-year-old female presents with symmetrical PIP joint pain and swelling in both hands. She complains of morning stiffness.

## Skin and soft tissue manifestations of rheumatological disease

a.   Pyoderma gangrenosum.          e.   Pannus.
b.   Keratoderma blennorrhagica.     f.   Dactylitis.
c.   Rheumatoid nodules.             g.   Erythema nodosum.
d.   Tophus.                         h.   Sclerodactyly.

Match the description of the patient with the most likely diagnosis.

11)   A 47-year-old female complains of dry eyes and a dry mouth. On examination, she has tender red nodules on both of her shins.

12)   A 67-year-old male is seen at his primary care doctor for an annual health check-up. His doctor notices a nodule on his right elbow; some of the skin overlying it is broken revealing a white, chalky appearance of the underlying tissue.

13)   A 24-year-old male who complains of joint pains and swelling is noted to have a waxy, yellow-brown, pustular rash on the soles of his feet.

14)   A 63-year-old female has a small, 2cm fibrous swelling over her left elbow joint.

15)   A 45-year-old female with rheumatoid arthritis develops a painful enlarging ulcer on her shin which is purple around the edges.

## Side effects of rheumatology drugs

a.   Colchicine.
b.   Naproxen.
c.   Ciclosporin.
d.   Methotrexate.

e.   Hydroxychloroquine.
f.   Etanercept.
g.   Sulfasalazine.
h.   Prednisolone.

Match each drug with the possible side effects seen in each patient.

16) A male being treated for gout develops profuse diarrhoea and nausea.

17) A female on therapy for rheumatoid arthritis complains of easy bruising and mouth ulcers.

18) A patient with a positive Mantoux test is unable to have this drug.

19) A patient being treated for rheumatoid arthritis complains of poor wound healing and weight gain.

20) A male develops a gastric ulcer secondary to intake of this drug.

# Vasculitis

a. Henoch-Schönlein purpura (HSP).
b. Takayasu's arteritis.
c. Polymyalgia rheumatica.
d. Goodpasture's disease

e. Wegener's disease
f. Polyarteritis nodosum.
g. Giant cell arteritis.
h. Behçet's disease.

Match the description of the patient with the most likely diagnosis.

21) A 30-year-old female complains of fever and malaise and later develops arm claudication with absent pulses and hypertension.

22) A Turkish male presents with painful oral and genital ulcers.

23) A male with chronic sinusitis and arthritis develops haemoptysis.

24) An 18-year-old girl complains of pain in her ankles and knees and a purpuric rash on her legs and thighs.

25) A 70-year-old male presents with a right-sided headache, flu-like symptoms and double vision.

## Autoantibodies

| | | | |
|---|---|---|---|
| a. | c-ANCA. | e. | Anti-Jo 1. |
| b. | Anti-Ro. | f. | Anti-Scl70. |
| c. | Anti-GBM. | g. | Anti-nuclear antibody (ANA). |
| d. | Anti-centromere antibody. | h. | Anti-dsDNA. |

Match the description of the disease with the most likely autoantibody.

26) Has the highest sensitivity in SLE.

27) Associated with Wegener's granulomatosis.

28) Can cause congenital heart block.

29) Found in Goodpasture's syndrome.

30) Positive in most patients with CREST syndrome.

## Causes of muscular pain

| | | | |
|---|---|---|---|
| a. | Polymyalgia rheumatica. | e. | Fibromyalgia. |
| b. | Polymyositis. | f. | Chronic fatigue syndrome. |
| c. | Dermatomyositis. | g. | SLE. |
| d. | Mixed connective tissue. | h. | Systemic sclerosis. |

Match the description of the patient with the most likely diagnosis.

31) A 32-year-old complains of unrefreshing sleep and widespread pain. She is tender to palpation in multiple sites in her neck, shoulders, buttocks and hips.

32) A 45-year-old female complains of shoulder weakness and fever. She is finding it increasingly difficult to raise her arm and she has difficulty climbing stairs.

33) A 45-year-old female describes widespread muscle aches and fatigue. She has experienced intermittent fever, widespread lymphadenopathy and recent weight loss. You notice a rash on her cheeks and nose.

34) A 70-year-old male complains of pain and stiffness in his shoulders and neck. This is worse on waking and improves throughout the morning.

35) A 20-year-old female presents with a 6-month debilitating fatigue and malaise. She has widespread muscular aches, tender lymph nodes to palpation and headaches. Her symptoms started after the death of her brother.

# First-line treatments in rheumatological disease

a.  NSAIDs.
b.  Nifedipine.
c.  IV methylprednisolone.
d.  Oral prednisolone.

e.  Hydroxychloroquine.
f.  Methotrexate.
g.  Sulfasalazine.
h.  Azathioprine.

Match the description with the most appropriate first-line treatment.

36) Is used to treat skin rashes seen in SLE.

37) A 21-year-old with lower back pain is diagnosed with ankylosing spondylitis.

38) DMARDs are used first-line to treat rheumatoid arthritis.

39) Used to treat Raynaud's phenomenon.

40) A 70-year-old male presenting with headache and blurred vision is diagnosed with giant cell arteritis (GCA).

## Cardiovascular complications of rheumatological disease

a.  Myocardial infarction.
b.  Libman-Sacks endocarditis.
c.  Aortic regurgitation.
d.  Dressler's syndrome.

e.  Coronary artery aneurysm.
f.  Aortic stenosis.
g.  Pulmonary hypertension.
h.  Pericarditis.

Match the description of the patient with the most likely diagnosis.

41) A 33-year-old male with longstanding ankylosing spondylitis develops shortness of breath. On examination, you detect a diastolic murmur best heard along the right sternal border.

42) A 24-year-old male recently diagnosed with reactive arthritis develops sharp left-sided chest pain. An ECG shows ST elevation in leads V2-6, I-III, aVF and aVL.

43) A 56-year-old female with a history of SLE is noted to have a new heart murmur. She undergoes an echocardiogram which demonstrates lesions on the mitral valve.

44) A 63-year-old female with systemic sclerosis develops an insidious onset of shortness of breath. On examination, you note a loud P2 of the second heart sound.

45) A 4-year-old boy is diagnosed with Kawasaki disease. He undergoes an echocardiogram which reveals this common cardiovascular complication.

# Short answer questions

1) A 27-year-old female presents with a 3-month history of fatigue, joint stiffness and pain worse on waking up. She has no past medical history of note. You observe a rash across the bridge of her nose, which is intensely itchy and spares the nasolabial folds. After taking a thorough investigation, you suspect SLE.

   a. Name two autoantibodies that may be present.    2 marks
   b. Give six other symptoms that she may mention.    3 marks
   c. What topical treatment could you suggest to improve her skin rash    1 mark
      and reduce flares of the disease?
   d. What oral medication could be used to treat her skin rash?    2 marks
   e. Six months later, she is noted to have an ejection systolic murmur.    2 marks
      What complication has she developed?

2) A 75-year-old male presents to his primary care doctor with a sudden onset of headache. The headache is worse on the right side and if he touches the area. He reports feeling generally unwell for the past 2 months, with fever and weight loss of 5kg. He has a past medical history of hypertension and osteoarthritis. His doctor requests further investigation for giant cell arteritis.

   a. Name two important symptoms that should be asked about.    2 marks
   b. Specify three features that may be found on examination.    3 marks
   c. What biochemical abnormality may be present?    1 mark
   d. What investigation could help confirm the diagnosis?    2 marks
   e. Name two pharmacological treatments that should be given.    2 marks

3) A 45-year-old female complains of a 3-month history of stiffness and pain in the MCP joints of her hands and intermittent swelling of her left wrist. Her past medical history includes depression. There is no family history of note. She works as a secretary and feels that this is interfering with her job as she is finding it increasingly difficult to type. After further investigation she is diagnosed with rheumatoid arthritis.

a. If this patient tests negative for rheumatoid factor, what other autoantibody could be checked? **2 marks**

b. Name four changes that may be seen in the hands and wrists of patients with rheumatoid arthritis. **4 marks**

c. What is the first-line disease-modifying anti-rheumatic drug in rheumatoid arthritis? **1 mark**

d. What should be prescribed with this medication? **1 mark**

e. What haematological abnormality is most likely to be seen on examination of this patient's full blood count? **2 marks**

4) A 67-year-old male presents with aching and weakness in his shoulders and back. He has lost 4kg over the past 8 weeks and complains of generalised malaise. On examination, he has scaly papules over the MCP joints of both hands. A diagnosis of dermatomyositis is suspected.

a. What is the name of the scaly papular rash described above and which is characteristic of dermatomyositis? **1 mark**

b. State two other skin changes associated with this condition. **2 marks**

c. Which enzyme is classically raised in dermatomyositis? **2 marks**

d. Name three other symptoms of this condition. **3 marks**

e. What is the first-line treatment in dermatomyositis? **2 marks**

5) A 35-year-old female with a past medical history of depression and anxiety attends the rheumatology clinic with a history of widespread body pain and fatigue. Although the pain has been present for several years, it has become worse in the last few months. On questioning, she reveals she is going through a stressful separation with her partner and is struggling to care for their two children. You suspect a diagnosis of fibromyalgia.

a. Name four other symptoms that she might complain of. 4 marks
b. Specify two non-pharmacological treatments that may help her symptoms. 1 mark
c. Aside from simple analgesia, what pharmacological treatment may relieve symptoms? 1 mark
d. Name three health professionals who may have a role in her care in a multidisciplinary team approach. 3 marks
e. Give two factors from her history that are linked to the development of fibromyalgia. 1 mark

6) A 19-year-old male who has recently returned from a gap year in Thailand presents to his primary care doctor with pain in his right knee and left ankle. He feels generally unwell and feverish and complains of itchy, red eyes. He mentions that 2 days before he flew back home he suffered from a bout of food poisoning. You suspect a diagnosis of reactive arthritis.

a. Name the third part of Reiter's triad, not noted above. 1 mark
b. Give two skin changes he may experience. 1 mark
c. Name four enteric organisms responsible for his symptoms. 4 marks
d. Specify one cardiovascular complication of this condition. 2 marks
e. What is the most likely outcome from this presentation? 2 marks

7)  A 63-year-old male presents with pain and swelling in the joints of his wrists and hands. He is generally fit and well but was diagnosed with psoriasis 5 years ago, which is controlled with emollient cream and topical steroids for flare-ups. On examination, you notice swelling in the DIP joints of both hands. He is diagnosed with psoriatic arthritis.

a.  Give three other changes that you might see on his hands.  3 marks
b.  Name three radiological features on an X-ray of his hands.  3 marks
c.  What is the most severe form of psoriatic arthritis called?  1 mark
d.  Name two DMARDs that can be used to treat this condition.  2 marks
e.  What biological therapy could be used if DMARDs were ineffective?  1 mark

8)  A 25-year-old male presents to his primary care doctor with an insidious onset of lower back pain. The pain is worse in the mornings and gets better throughout the day. He complains of a generalised malaise but no other symptoms. A diagnosis of ankylosing spondylitis is made.

a.  Which HLA type is associated with this condition?  1 mark
b.  Specify four extra-articular features he may experience.  4 marks
c.  What is the first-line management of this condition?  2 marks
d.  Name two radiological features that may be seen on X-ray.  2 marks
e.  What neurological consequence may occur with severe longstanding disease?  1 mark

9) A 45-year-old male presents to his primary care doctor with a persistent cough and recent episodes of haemoptysis. He complains of fever and night sweats, a hoarse voice and chronic sinusitis. He is otherwise fit and well. He has never smoked. His doctor is concerned about malignancy but after thorough investigation he is diagnosed with granulomatosis with polyangiitis (Wegener's granulomatosis).

a. Name six other symptoms that this man may complain of.          3 marks
b. What anatomical abnormality may cause his hoarse voice?          2 marks
c. Give two features you might see on examination of his face.          2 marks
d. What autoantibody is characteristic of this disease?          1 mark
e. Which drug is used to promote remission of the disease?          2 marks

10) A 62-year-old obese male presents with a hot, swollen, painful 1st MTP joint. He has a background of Type 2 diabetes mellitus with Stage 2 chronic kidney disease, hypertension and hyperlipidaemia. His medications include metformin, ramipril, simvastatin, amlodipine and sildenafil. He drinks approximately 40 units of alcohol per week. You suspect a diagnosis of gout. A joint aspiration is taken for examination.

a. What would you see on microscopy which would confirm a diagnosis of gout?          2 marks
b. What biochemical abnormality is likely to be present that would contribute to his presentation?          2 marks
c. What treatment could you offer him during this attack?          1 mark
d. On examination, you notice a chalky nodule on his right ear. What complication has he developed?          2 marks
e. Give three things you could advise him to reduce his risk of further attacks.          3 marks

11) A 27-year-old female presents with an insidious onset of pain in her wrist and PIP joints of both hands. She complains of debilitating fatigue and has dropped two dress sizes in the past 6 months without any deliberate weight loss. She smokes approximately 20 cigarettes a day, drinks 30 units of alcohol a week and is currently unemployed. She has no past medical history of note. You suspect a diagnosis of rheumatoid arthritis.

a. What HLA type is rheumatoid arthritis associated with? 2 marks

b. Two months later she develops numbness and tingling in her right 2 marks lateral three digits of the hand. What complication has she developed?

c. Name one feature in her history which is associated with a worse 2 marks prognosis in rheumatoid arthritis.

d. What scoring system can be used to measure disease activity in 2 marks rheumatoid arthritis?

e. She is given a trial of two different DMARDs with little effect. A 2 marks decision is made to start her on a TNF-alpha inhibitor. Give an example of a drug that might be used.

12) A 62-year-old male with a history of chronic kidney disease, hypertension and diabetes presents with an acutely tender and swollen right knee. He is pyrexial with a raised WCC but is haemodynamically stable with no systemic symptoms. After investigation, a diagnosis of pseudogout is made.

a. What investigation should be performed to exclude a diagnosis of 2 marks septic arthritis?

b. What is the composition of the crystals in pseudogout? 2 marks

c. Give three risk factors for pseudogout. 3 marks

d. What might be seen on joint X-ray? 2 marks

e. What can you tell him about the likely time course for this acute 1 mark attack?

13) A 43-year-old male presents with a 2-month history of wheeze and shortness of breath which is increasing in severity. He complains of recurrent sinusitis and fatigue. On examination, you note nasal polyps and a scattered wheeze. A chest X-ray shows pulmonary infiltrates. You refer him for investigation of Churg-Strauss syndrome (eosinophilic granulomatosis with polyangiitis).

a.  What abnormality seen on blood tests is part of the diagnostic criteria     2 marks
    for Churg-Strauss syndrome?
b.  Give two other abnormalities found on blood testing in Churg-Strauss     2 marks
    syndrome.
c.  Which autoantibody may be present?     1 mark
d.  Give four complications of the disease.     4 marks
e.  What is the first-line treatment for this disease?     1 mark

# Chapter 9

# Infectious disease
## QUESTIONS

## Single best answer questions

1) A 28-year-old male presents to his primary care doctor feeling generally unwell complaining of a fever, muscle aches and a sore throat. On examination, he has pharyngitis and widespread lymphadenopathy. On further questioning he had unprotected sexual intercourse 4 weeks ago with another male. What is the most likely diagnosis?

a. Secondary syphilis.
b. EBV infection.
c. HIV seroconversion.
d. *Cytomegalovirus* infection.

2) A 34-year-old Indian male presents to his primary care doctor complaining of visual disturbance. He has noticed progressively worsening blurriness particularly in the centre of his vision; he does not complain of any pain or eye redness. He was commenced on an antibiotic regime 2 months ago for TB. Which is the most likely cause of his symptoms?

a. Rifampicin.
b. Isoniazid.
c. Pyrazinamide.
d. Ethambutol.

3) A 72-year-old female presents to the emergency department with a 2-day history of headache, myalgia, dry cough and fever. She reports loose stools 4 days ago which have now resolved and has recently been on holiday to Spain. On examination, she is pyrexial and appears mildly confused. Her blood results show she is hyponatraemic and there is bi-basal consolidation present on her chest X-ray. What is the most likely causative organism?

a. *Streptococcus pneumoniae.*
b. *Mycoplasma pneumoniae.*
c. *Legionella pneumophila.*
d. *Haemophilus influenzae.*

4) An 18-year-old student who has recently moved over from India to start university presents to her primary care doctor with a severe sore throat and swollen neck. On examination, she has a low-grade pyrexia, there is a grey pseudomembrane covering the pharynx and tonsils, and there is significant tender cervical lymphadenopathy. What is the most likely diagnosis?

a.   Diphtheria.
b.   Epiglottitis.
c.   Streptococcal pharyngitis.
d.   Mumps.

5) A 23-year-old female presents with a 2-day history of jaundice and abdominal pain preceded by feeling generally unwell with anorexia and malaise. She reports a recent holiday to Egypt where she enjoyed the local food. Since her holiday she reports she has stopped smoking as she has lost the taste for it. Given the most likely diagnosis, how is this infection most commonly transmitted?

a.   Faecal-oral transmission.
b.   Vertical transmission.
c.   Droplet transmission.
d.   Blood transmission.

6) A 17-year-old female presents very unwell to the emergency department with a fever of 39°, tachycardia, a diffuse macular rash and hypotension refractory to fluid resuscitation. According to her mother she is usually fit and well, she is currently menstruating and normally uses tampons. She is admitted to the intensive care unit for cardiovascular support and is commenced on IV antibiotics. Clinically she starts to improve after several days at which point it is noticed that the skin on her palms and soles is peeling off. What is the most likely diagnosis?

a.  Meningococcal septicaemia.
b.  Toxic shock syndrome.
c.  Scalded skin syndrome.
d.  Toxic epidermal necrolysis.

7) A 33-year-old alcoholic presents to the emergency department with a productive cough and pyrexia. On examination, he looks unkempt and you can smell alcohol. His blood tests show raised inflammatory markers and his chest X-ray shows left upper lobe consolidation. What is the most likely causative organism of his pneumonia?

a.  *Streptococcus pneumoniae.*
b.  *Mycoplasma pneumoniae.*
c.  *Klebsiella pneumoniae.*
d.  *Chlamydia psittaci.*

8) A 23-year-old female is on her gap year in Thailand and she attends the emergency department in Bangkok complaining of a severe headache, pain behind her eyes and generalised muscle aches. On examination, she is pyrexial and has a positive tourniquet test. You suspect

dengue fever. Which signs on examination would concern you that she has severe dengue fever?

a. Ascites.
b. Positive tourniquet test.
c. Mucosal bleeding.
d. Impaired conscious level.

9) A 19-year-old sexually active female presents to the emergency department acutely unwell with sudden-onset fever, rigors and severe back pain associated with vomiting. On examination, she looks unwell and has significant tenderness over her left costovertebral angle. She grows *Escherichia coli* in her urine culture. What is the most likely diagnosis?

a. Ectopic pregnancy.
b. Acute pyelonephritis.
c. Pelvic inflammatory disease.
d. Cystitis.

10) An 8-year-old child with known sickle cell disease is brought to the emergency department with right thigh pain and swelling. He undergoes multiple investigations which show osteomyelitis. What is the most likely causative organism?

a. *Salmonella spp.*
b. *Streptococcus pyogenes.*
c. *Staphylococcus epidermidis.*
d. *Staphylococcus aureus.*

11) A 38-year-old HIV-positive intravenous drug user attends the emergency department with increasing confusion and agitation over the last 3 days and had a seizure this morning. He has poor compliance with his anti-retroviral medications and has failed to attend multiple clinic appointments. A CT of the head shows multiple ring-enhancing lesions. What is the likely diagnosis?

a.  Progressive multifocal leukoencephalopathy.
b.  Cerebral toxoplasmosis.
c.  Brain abscess.
d.  Cryptococcal meningitis.

12) A 28-year-old female who has recently returned from rural Africa presents to the emergency department with fever, headache and myalgia. Whilst waiting to be reviewed she has a generalised tonic-clonic seizure. You suspect this could be cerebral malaria. Which of the *Plasmodium spp.* is the most likely cause?

a.  *Plasmodium vivax.*
b.  *Plasmodium malariae.*
c.  *Plasmodium falciparum.*
d.  *Plasmodium ovale.*

13) A 29-year-old HIV-positive intravenous drug user is seen in the clinic. She reports visual changes with floaters and blurriness. She is non-compliant with medications and has a CD4 count of 47. You perform fundoscopy and find pizza pie changes. What is the most likely cause of her symptoms?

a. *Herpes simplex* virus.
b. *Cryptococcus spp.*
c. *Cytomegalovirus.*
d. *Mycobacterium tuberculosis.*

14) A 24-year-old male has had a splenectomy following a road traffic accident. It is explained that he is now at risk of overwhelming sepsis from encapsulated organisms and requires life-long antibiotic prophylaxis. He has no known drug allergies. Which one of the following would you prescribe first-line?

a. Doxycycline.
b. Metronidazole.
c. Gentamicin.
d. Penicillin V.

15) A 23-year-old female has recently returned to the UK following 6 months of travelling. She attends her primary care doctor with a 10-day history of feeling generally unwell, associated with a headache, occasional non-specific abdominal pain and constipation. She has attended today as she is concerned about a rash she has developed. On examination, you note rose spots on her abdomen. What is the most likely diagnosis?

a. Malaria.
b. Typhoid fever.
c. Dengue fever.
d. Leptospirosis.

16) A 29-year-old male attends the genitourinary medicine clinic concerned regarding a genital ulcer he has developed following unprotected sexual intercourse 2 weeks prior. On examination, you note a chancre and moderate lymphadenopathy. IM benzyl penicillin is given empirically to treat primary syphilis, but 2 hours later he develops a fever, headache, myalgia and rigors. What is the most likely cause of these symptoms?

a. Sepsis.
b. Drug-related reaction.
c. HIV seroconversion.
d. Jarisch-Herxheimer reaction.

17) A 36-year-old female is brought to the emergency department by her husband. She has been off work for a week with influenza. He is concerned as she doesn't seem to be improving and since this morning has been very breathless. On examination, she is pyrexial, tachypnoeic, tachycardic and hypotensive. She has bilateral coarse crackles on auscultation and her chest X-ray shows bilateral consolidation with cavitation. What is the most likely causative organism?

a. *Staphylococcus aureus.*
b. *Streptococcus pneumoniae.*
c. *Mycoplasma pneumoniae.*
d. *Klebsiella pneumoniae.*

18) A 19-year-old male is brought by ambulance to the emergency department following a seizure at home. His mother has accompanied him and she reports he has been acting strangely over the last couple of days with increasing confusion and has complained of a headache. Prior to this he was fit and well with no history of seizures. On examination, he is pyrexial at 38.9° and disorientated to time and place. What is the most likely diagnosis?

a. Meningitis.
b. Encephalitis.
c. Space-occupying lesion.
d. Epilepsy.

19) A mother brings her 2-year-old in to see her primary care doctor with non-bloody diarrhoea, abdominal pain and fever. The child is normally fit and well and is up to date with her immunisations. The mother reports several similar cases in the nursery that her child normally attends. What is the most likely cause of this child's gastroenteritis?

a. Rotavirus.
b. *Salmonella spp.*
c. *Escherichia coli O157.*
d. Norovirus.

20) An 8-year-old child is admitted to hospital with haemolytic uraemic syndrome which developed following a diarrhoeal illness suspected to be *E. coli O157*. Haemolytic uraemic syndrome is a triad of microangiopathic haemolytic anaemia, acute kidney injury and which one of the following?

a.   Fever.
b.   Raised WCC.
c.   Thrombocytopenia.
d.   Bloody diarrhoea.

21) An 80-year-old female is treated for pneumonia with two prolonged courses of antibiotics. She develops profuse watery diarrhoea, severe abdominal pain and signs of shock. Her WCC is raised at $22.0 \times 10^9$/L. What would you expect to see on an abdominal X-ray?

a.   Toxic megacolon.
b.   Lead-pipe colon.
c.   Faecal loading.
d.   Coffee-bean sign.

22) Which one of the following causes of viral hepatitis is unusual in that it cannot occur in the absence of hepatitis B virus?

a.   Hepatitis A.
b.   Hepatitis C.
c.   Hepatitis D.
d.   Hepatitis E.

23) A researcher is keen to explore the role of insects in vector-borne diseases and decides to study human African trypanosomiasis, also known as African sleeping sickness. Which one of the following is the disease vector for African sleeping sickness?

a. Anopheles mosquitos.
b. Sandflies.
c. Ticks.
d. Tsetse fies.

# Extended matching questions

## Lumbar puncture interpretation

a.  Bacterial meningitis.
b.  Subarachnoid haemorrhage.
c.  Multiple sclerosis.
d.  Idiopathic intracranial hypertension.

e.  Viral meningitis.
f.  Sarcoidosis.
g.  Guillain-Barré syndrome.
h.  TB meningitis.

Match the lumbar puncture results to the most likely diagnosis.

1)  Turbid CSF, 1250/mm³ WCC, 95% polymorphonuclear leukocytes, low glucose level.

2)  Clear CSF, 5/mm³ WCC, protein 0.60g/L, IgG oligoclonal bands.

3)  Clear CSF, 80/mm³ WCC, protein 0.48g/L, 88% lymphocytes, normal glucose level.

4)  Clear CSF, 2/mm³ WCC, 1 RBC, normal protein, normal glucose, opening pressure raised at 30cm H₂O.

5)  Opaque CSF, fibrin web, 150/mm³ WCC, 85% lymphocytes, protein 1.60g/L.

## Loose stools

| | |
|---|---|
| a. | *Vibrio cholera.* |
| b. | *E. coli O517.* |
| c. | *Clostridium difficile.* |
| d. | Rotavirus. |

| | |
|---|---|
| e. | *Giardia lamblia.* |
| f. | *Bacillus cereus.* |
| g. | *Staphylococcus aureus.* |
| h. | *Campylobacter jejuni.* |

Match the organism to the cause of the patient's loose stools.

6) An 18-year-old develops diarrhoea after reheating rice from a takeaway.

7) A 24-year-old female develops profuse, 'rice-water' stools following a recent holiday to India.

8) A 6-year-old visits a farm on a school trip. He later develops bloody loose stools and ends up admitted to hospital where he is found to have a low haemoglobin, raised bilirubin and an acute kidney injury.

9) A 47-year-old male develops leg weakness. On examination, he has absent ankle reflexes. He reports a diarrhoeal illness 2 weeks previously.

10) A 26-year-old male develops profuse, explosive vomiting 2 hours after eating a takeaway. Twenty-four hours later he feels completely back to normal.

## Infective causes of jaundice

| | | | | |
|---|---|---|---|---|
| a. | Hepatitis A. | | e. | EBV. |
| b. | Hepatitis B. | | f. | Schistosomiasis. |
| c. | Hepatitis C. | | g. | Malaria. |
| d. | Leptospirosis. | | h. | *Cytomegalovirus.* |

Match the description to the most likely infective cause of jaundice.

11) A 28-year-old sewage worker presents to the emergency department with a flu-like illness and jaundice. His admission bloods show an acute kidney injury.

12) A 17-year-old complains of a severe sore throat and myalgia. She was given a course of amoxicillin from which she developed a widespread rash. She is mildly jaundiced, with splenomegaly, pharyngitis and cervical lymphadenopathy.

13) Thick and thin blood smears can be used to diagnose this.

14) A 48-year-old ex-intravenous drug user with chronic hepatitis is diagnosed with Sjögren's syndrome.

15) A 23-year-old female attends her primary care doctor after getting back from holiday in South-East Asia complaining of malaise, anorexia and mild jaundice. She has stopped smoking since returning as she "hasn't felt the cravings".

# Pneumonia

| | | | |
|---|---|---|---|
| a. | *Streptococcus pneumoniae.* | e. | *Legionella pneumophila.* |
| b. | *Klebsiella pneumoniae.* | f. | *Pseudomonas aeruginosa.* |
| c. | *Mycoplasma pneumoniae.* | g. | *Pneumocystis jirovecii.* |
| d. | *Staphylococcus aureus.* | h. | *Chlamydophila psittaci.* |

## Match the description to the most likely cause of pneumonia.

16) Gram-negative rod that commonly colonises cystic fibrosis patients.

17) An important cause of atypical pneumonia that should be considered if the patient has been exposed to sick birds.

18) This organism most commonly causes community-acquired pneumonia.

19) Associated with target lesions.

20) A common cause of pneumonia after a viral infection such as influenza and measles.

## Childhood infections

| | | | |
|---|---|---|---|
| a. | Whooping cough. | e. | Mumps. |
| b. | Measles. | f. | Rubella. |
| c. | Epiglottitis. | g. | Scarlet fever. |
| d. | Slapped cheek syndrome. | h. | Croup. |

Match the description to the most likely childhood infection.

21) Prodrome of cough, coryza, conjunctivitis and Koplik spots.

22) Presents with a toxic looking child, severe sore throat and drooling as they are unable to swallow saliva. May have respiratory distress and stridor.

23) Has a rash with a texture that may feel like sandpaper.

24) Usually caused by *Bordetella pertussis*, a known risk factor for developing bronchiectasis later in life.

25) Most commonly caused by the parainfluenza virus. It may present with a barking cough and in some cases stridor.

# Antibiotics

| | | | |
|---|---|---|---|
| a. | Gentamicin. | e. | Clarithromycin. |
| b. | Amoxicillin. | f. | Ceftriaxone. |
| c. | Metronidazole. | g. | Ciprofloxacin. |
| d. | Vancomycin. | h. | Cefuroxime. |

## Match the description to the correct antimicrobial agent.

26) A glycopeptide antibiotic used in severe *Clostridium difficile* infection.

27) A third-generation cephalosporin useful in meningitis due to its ability to cross the blood-brain barrier.

28) Effective against anaerobes, but patients are advised not to drink alcohol.

29) A macrolide antibiotic used alongside co-amoxiclav in severe community-acquired pneumonia.

30) A fluoroquinolone antibiotic, it has good action against Gram-negative bacteria and should not be prescribed for patients with epilepsy.

## Infections of the central nervous system

a.   *Listeria monocytogenes.*          e.   Brain abscess.

b.   *Neisseria meningitidis.*          f.   Group B *Streptococcus.*

c.   *Herpes simplex.*                  g.   Rabies.

d.   *Cryptococcus.*                    h.   Malaria.

## Match the description to the most likely cause of CNS infection.

31)   Found in immunosuppressed patients. Indian ink stain is used to aid diagnosis under microscopy.

32)   Associated with ingestion of soft cheeses. Ampicillin is added when this is suspected.

33)   A 12-year-old child presents unwell with meningitis. Gram-negative diplococci are seen on examination of CSF.

34)   A cause of new-born meningitis, often carried asymptomatically by women in the vagina.

35)   CT imaging shows a ring-enhancing lesion.

## Genito-urinary infections

a. Bacterial vaginosis.
b. *Chlamydia trachomatis.*
c. *Trichomonas vaginalis.*
d. Genital warts.

e. Genital herpes.
f. *Neisseria gonorrhoeae.*
g. Primary syphilis.
h. Vaginal thrush.

Match the description to the most likely genito-urinary infection.

36) A 24-year-old female complains of frothy greenish-yellow, smelly vaginal discharge. On examination, she has a strawberry cervix appearance.

37) Caused by a Gram-negative diplococcus.

38) Treated with metronidazole. Clue cells are found on microscopy.

39) Intracellular Gram-negative bacteria and commonly asymptomatic in females.

40) The incidence of this genito-urinary infection has decreased since the introduction of the HPV screening programme.

## Opportunistic infections

a.  Kaposi's sarcoma.                         e.  Oesophageal candidiasis.
b.  *Mycobacterium avium* complex.  f.  *Cytomegalovirus.*
c.  *Pneumocystis jirovecii.*            g.  Toxoplasmosis.
d.  *Cryptosporidium.*                     h.  Cervical cancer.

Match the description to the condition or causative organism found in patients with human immunodeficiency virus and low CD4 counts.

41) Causes a retinitis which on fundoscopy shows classical pizza pie changes.

42) Can cause severe diarrhoea leading to weight loss. Patients tend to be otherwise well with no abdominal pain or fever.

43) Presents with odynophagia and usually responds well to fluconazole.

44) Caused by human *Herpes* virus 8.

45) Causes a respiratory infection. Patients classically desaturate on exertion.

## Short answer questions

1) A 72-year-old male presents to the emergency department with a 3-day history of a cough productive of green sputum, shortness of breath and fever. He is normally fit and well with a past medical history of hypertension. He smokes 10 cigarettes per day, has no known drug allergies and takes ramipril 5mg od. On examination, he has a temperature of 38.6°C, his respiratory rate is 32 breaths per minute, he is disorientated and coarse crackles are heard on auscultation of the right lung base. You suspect he has community-acquired pneumonia and take a full set of bloods including cultures.

a. Name two bacterial organisms that can commonly cause community-acquired pneumonia (genus and species).  2 marks

b. Give three other investigations that would be appropriate in investigating community-acquired pneumonia.  3 marks

c. Give an appropriate score to predict severity and aid the management of community-acquired pneumonia.  1 mark

d. Using the above score you decide this is a severe pneumonia. Name two antibiotics that this patient should be prescribed.  2 marks

e. Give two complications of community-acquired pneumonia.  2 marks

2) A 19-year-old university student presents to his primary care doctor complaining of a several-day history of fever, sore throat, malaise and severe fatigue. On examination, he has palpable cervical lymphadenopathy, pharyngitis and you are able to palpate a mass in the left side of his abdomen. You clinically diagnose infectious mononucleosis.

a. You suspect that the abdominal mass is most likely an enlarged spleen. Give two examination findings that would confirm it is a palpable spleen and not his kidney.   2 marks

b. You take some routine blood tests and a rapid test for Epstein-Barr virus (EBV). What is the rapid test that has been taken?   2 marks

c. His blood results come back; his blood film demonstrates an abnormality of his white blood cells and his liver function tests are mildly deranged. What abnormality of his white blood cells is likely to have been visualised?   2 marks

d. Give three viral causes of the above presentation other than EBV.   3 marks

e. He is keen to restart playing rugby. What would you advise him about playing contact sports?   1 mark

3) A 28-year-old intravenous drug user presents to the emergency department complaining of a non-productive cough, fever and progressive shortness of breath. On examination, he looks unkempt and is cachectic. His temperature is 38.1°C, his oxygen saturation is 92% on air and drops to 87% when he walks to the toilet. On examination of his chest, he has bibasal crepitations and a scattered wheeze, and his chest X-ray shows bibasal pulmonary infiltrates. You perform an arterial blood gas.

| | |
|---|---|
| pH | 7.35 (7.35-7.45) |
| $pO_2$ | 7.8 (10-14kPa) |
| $pCO_2$ | 4.6 (4.5-6kPa) |
| Base excess | -1 (-2-2mmol/L) |
| $HCO_3^-$ | 22 (22-26mmol/L) |

a. What abnormality is demonstrated on the above ABG?    2 marks

b. What is the most likely causative organism?    2 marks

c. You suspect the patient may have an underlying HIV infection. Give    4 marks
four other AIDS-defining illnesses.

d. What antibiotic would you commence in this patient?    1 mark

e. The patient is followed up after discharge; he is commenced on highly    1 mark
active anti-retroviral therapy. His viral load and a cell count are being
monitored. Which cell count is this?

4) A 34-year-old female presents to the emergency
department complaining of poor oral intake, fever and
worsening right upper quadrant pain. She returned from
travelling around Asia approximately 3 months ago.
Whilst away she had a short period of abdominal pain and
bloody, loose stools; however, this self-resolved. On
examination, she is pyrexial at 37.9°C and has tender
hepatomegaly, she looks pale but there are no signs of
jaundice.

a. What is the most likely underlying organism?    2 marks

b. What is the most likely cause of the abdominal pain?    2 marks

c. Specify four blood tests you would request and explain the rationale    4 marks
for choosing these tests.

d. What imaging would you request to initially investigate the    1 mark
abdominal pain?

e. Give one piece of advice you would give to patients travelling abroad    1 mark
to reduce the risk of catching this condition.

5) A 37-year-old male of Mediterranean origin presents to the emergency department pyrexial with a headache and myalgia after recently returning from a year-long volunteering trip to Africa. Whilst away he was diagnosed with malaria which he states was treated with a monotherapy of an anti-malarial drug; he completed this course 6 months ago. He has a past medical history of a haematological condition which means he is unable to take certain medications including sulphonamides and nitrofurantoin but is otherwise fit and well. He has no regular medications and no allergies.

a. You are keen to exclude malaria. What is the gold standard investigation you would request to confirm the diagnosis? **2 marks**

b. The above investigation comes back as positive for *Plasmodium vivax*. Why is *Plasmodium vivax* prone to reactivation following the initial infection? **3 marks**

c. You commence the patient on chloroquine and primaquine. He becomes jaundiced and develops back pain soon after commencing treatment. You suspect he may be having a haemolytic crisis. What is the most likely underlying haematological condition? **1 mark**

d. Give two interventions that you would advise a traveller to an endemic area to do to reduce their risk of contracting malaria. **2 marks**

e. Malaria is a notifiable illness. Give two other examples of notifiable diseases. **2 marks**

6) A concerned mother brings her 4-year-old child to the primary care doctor. The child has been complaining of a headache and mum reports that her child has been more lethargic and sleepier than normal. On examination, the child looks unwell, has cold hands and feet, and you notice a spreading, petechial rash. The child is normally fit and well, is up to date with all vaccinations and has no

known drug allergies. You arrange urgent admission to hospital as you are concerned the child may have meningococcal disease.

a.  What antibiotic should be administered whilst awaiting transfer to hospital and which route of administration should be used?    2 marks

b.  Name three components of the Glasgow Coma Scale.    3 marks

c.  Which six therapies make up the Sepsis Six bundle?    3 marks

d.  You perform a lumbar puncture which shows Gram-negative diplococci. What is the most likely causative organism?    1 mark

e.  Give one antibiotic for chemoprophylaxis in close contacts.    1 mark

7)  A 52-year-old male presents to his primary care doctor with progressive, non-specific symptoms including malaise and general fatigue. He has a past medical history of mild haemophilia and has had multiple blood transfusions over several different decades. He is otherwise normally fit and well. He takes no regular medications other than when he experiences an acute bleeding episode; he denies any recent episodes. He is a non-smoker and drinks half a bottle of wine per week. You order some investigations and the results are suggestive of chronic hepatitis C infection.

a.  Give two ways that hepatitis C can be transmitted.    2 marks

b.  Give eight blood tests that may be performed as part of a non-invasive liver screen.    4 marks

c.  You want to rule out a focal liver lesion. What first-line imaging would you order to assess this?    1 mark

d.  Give two parameters of the Child-Pugh score to assess prognosis of chronic liver disease.    2 marks

e.  What would you advise the patient with regards to alcohol consumption?    1 mark

8) A 52-year-old female presents to her primary care doctor with an acutely swollen, painful right knee. She feels feverish and generally unwell and her pain has progressed to the point where she is now unable to weight-bear. She has a past medical history of poorly controlled diabetes mellitus and hypertension. She has no known drug allergies and takes metformin, insulin and ramipril. On examination, her temperature is 37.9°C and she is tachycardic, her knee is visibly swollen, very tender and has a reduced range of movement. You suspect she may have septic arthritis and she is admitted to hospital for further investigations.

a. What is the most likely causative organism?                                    1 mark

b. Give three differentials for a single acutely inflamed joint.                   3 marks

c. What investigation would you perform prior to commencing   1 mark
   antibiotics to confirm diagnosis?

d. What would you expect to see on examination of synovial fluid in:   4 marks
   i. Gout?
   ii. Pseudogout?

e. You suspect this patient's erratic blood sugars have contributed   1 mark
   towards the presentation. What blood test could you perform to
   assess her long-term glycaemic control?

9) A 23-year-old female is taken unwell on a flight home from India to the United Kingdom with severe, watery diarrhoea associated with nausea. Her parents take her straight from the airport to the emergency department; she collapses in the waiting room. On examination, she looks unwell and profoundly dehydrated. You immediately commence IV fluids and catheterise her to strictly monitor input and output.

a.   Give four findings on examination to indicate dehydration.          4 marks

b.   You obtain a stool sample which has a rice water appearance. What is   1 mark
     the most likely diagnosis?

c.   Whilst taking routine blood tests, you also take a venous blood gas.   2 marks
     What does the following blood gas show?

| | |
|---|---|
| pH | 7.28 (7.35-7.45) |
| $pO_2$ | 12.4 (10-14kPa) |
| $pCO_2$ | 3.8 (4.5-6kPa) |
| $HCO_3^-$ | 17 (22-26mmol/L) |

d.   What is the most common cause of travellers' diarrhoea?          1 mark

e.   Give two pieces of advice you would tell a patient going travelling to   2 marks
     reduce their risk of developing travellers' diarrhoea.

10)  An 88-year-old female has had a prolonged stay on the
     geriatric ward. She was initially admitted with a urinary tract
     infection. Following completion of antibiotics she developed
     a hospital-acquired pneumonia. She takes metformin,
     lansoprazole, amlodipine, bendroflumethiazide, paracetamol
     and aspirin. You are asked to see her as she has developed a
     low-grade pyrexia and watery diarrhoea which has a
     particularly unpleasant smell; she has opened her bowels
     six times overnight. You are concerned she may have
     developed a *Clostridium difficile* infection which she has not
     had previously.

a.   Give four points in the history suggestive of *Clostridium difficile* infection.   4 marks

b.   What visual guide can be used to classify the form of stool?          1 mark

c.   What would you commence if this was confirmed?          1 mark

d.   *Clostridium difficile* is confirmed and she does not respond to initial   2 marks
     treatment. What antibiotic would you now commence and via what
     route?

e.   State two physical measures that can be implemented to reduce the   2 marks
     risk of any other patients contracting the infection.

11) A 27-year-old male is seen in a primary care doctor outreach programme. He is a current intravenous drug user who moved into a hostel 3 months ago where he shares a bedroom with 9 other males. He has a background of hepatitis C and HIV infection for which he is poorly compliant with medication and hospital appointments. He complains of progressive weight loss, night sweats and haemoptysis, and reports similar symptoms in two of his room mates. You are highly suspicious that this patient has pulmonary tuberculosis and perform further investigations; he is smear-negative.

a. Give two risk factors in the above history for tuberculosis. 2 mark

b. The diagnosis is confirmed. He is commenced on four medications to treat his pulmonary tuberculosis. Match the newly commenced medication to the side effect that it can cause: 4 marks
i. Peripheral neuropathy.
ii. Red/orange urine.
iii. Optic neuritis.
iv. Gout.

c. You are concerned that due to his lifestyle he may not adhere to therapy. What can be used to confirm adherence? 1 mark

d. What test could you offer to his close contacts? 1 mark

e. What is the characteristic finding of TB on biopsy? 2 marks

12) A 19-year-old female attends a genitourinary medicine outpatient clinic for routine screening after having sexual intercourse with a new partner. She denies any symptoms. She has had two sexual partners in the last 12 months and intermittently uses barrier contraception; she has a contraceptive implant and experiences irregular, light vaginal bleeding due to this. She is normally fit and well, denies any past medical history, has had no previous sexually transmitted infections and has no known drug

allergies. You perform routine screening and results come back as positive for *Chlamydia*. She has no evidence of any other sexually transmitted infections and her pregnancy test is negative.

a. *Chlamydia* is commonly asymptomatic. Give four symptoms that a female patient may complain of. 4 marks

b. Give two signs that you may find on examination. 2 marks

c. What molecular technique is used to detect *Chlamydia*? 1 mark

d. Name an appropriate antibiotic for this patient's condition. 1 mark

e. Give two complications that can occur in women with untreated *Chlamydia* infection. 2 marks

13) A 54-year-old female presents to her primary care doctor with a burning pain on the left side of her chest. On examination, the altered sensation occurs in a single dermatomal pattern that does not cross the midline and you notice clusters of small vesicles which she says have only appeared today and are weeping. She has a past medical history of diabetes and on further questioning had chickenpox as a child and works as a school teacher. You believe she has shingles.

a. What is the underlying causative organism? 2 marks

b. Explain why shingles can reoccur after the initial infection. 2 marks

c. The patient would like to know: 2 marks
   i. Can she go to work following this appointment?
   ii. When will she no longer be infectious?

d. At follow-up 2 months later, the patient, following resolution, describes a burning pain in the affected area: 3 marks
   i. What is the most likely diagnosis?
   ii. Give two first-line medications that should be initially considered to manage neuropathic pain.

e. What is the eponymous name given to shingles causing ear pain, unilateral facial weakness and a change in taste sensation? 1 mark

# Section 2
# Answers

# Chapter 10

## Cardiology
### ANSWERS

1) b.
2) b.
3) a.
4) c.
5) c.
6) d.
7) a.
8) b.
9) c.
10) c.
11) b.
12) b.
13) a.
14) c.
15) b.
16) c.
17) b.
18) d.
19) c.
20) b.

21)  a.
22)  c.
23)  b.

# Extended matching question answers

1) h

This is an increase in pulse pressure >15mmHg on inspiration. It is associated with severe asthma and cardiac tamponade.

2) c

This is a characteristic finding in aortic stenosis.

3) a

This finding is characteristic for mixed valvular disease.

4) e

This is classic of mitral stenosis and is a palpable first heart sound.

5) b

A jerky pulse is quick and strong and is caused by vigorous contraction of the hypertrophic left ventricle.

6) a

NYHA I — no limitations.

7) d

NYHA IV — symptoms at rest. Any physical activity worsens symptoms.

8) b

NYHA II — slight limitations. Comfortable at rest, but ordinary physical activity results in fatigue, palpations, dyspnoea or pain.

9)  c

NYHA III — marked limitations. Mild activity leads to symptoms.

10)  c

NYHA III — marked limitations. Mild activity leads to symptoms.

11)  b

The common side effects of adenosine include: a sense of impending doom, bronchospasm, headache and AV block.

12)  e

The common side effects of loop diuretics include: tinnitus, AKI, dizziness and gout.

13)  g

The common side effects of amiodarone include: thyroid dysfunction, deranged liver function, lung fibrosis and slate-coloured skin.

14)  h

The common side effects of aspirin include: bleeding, gastritis and bronchospasm.

15)  c

The common side effects of ACE inhibitors include: a bothersome cough, AKI and flash pulmonary oedema.

16)  c

This is a pericarditis that occurs 2-6 weeks following an MI.

17)  d

This is an aneurysm that occurs 4-6 weeks following an MI. It can lead to recurrent ventricular tachycardia, left ventricular failure and systemic emboli.

18)  g

This is a thrombus that adheres to a blood vessel wall.


19)  h

This is due to a failure of the mitral valve.


20)  b

This is inflammation of the pericardium which occurs early following an MI. It causes a pleuritic chest pain that is relieved by sitting forward.


21)  a

The current NICE guideline for >55 years of age and/or Afro-Caribbean is to use a calcium channel blocker.


22)  g

The current NICE guideline for poorly controlled hypertension despite first-line treatment is to use a combination (ACE inhibitor and calcium channel blocker).


23)  d

The current NICE guideline for poorly controlled hypertension, despite combination therapy, is to use a thiazide-like diuretic adjunct.


24)  b

The current NICE guideline for hypertension in pregnancy is to use labetalol as the first-line medication.


25)  a

The current NICE guideline for >55 years of age and/or Afro-Caribbean is a calcium channel blocker.

26) c

Diastolic murmurs include: aortic regurgitation, mitral stenosis, pulmonary regurgitation (rare) and tricuspid stenosis (rare). A loud first heart sound is associated with mitral valve disorders.

27) d

Pansystolic murmurs are either tricuspid regurgitation or mitral regurgitation and left-sided murmurs are enhanced on expiration.

28) a

An ejection systolic murmur with radiation to the carotids is aortic stenosis (without radiation this is suggestive of aortic sclerosis).

29) e

Pansystolic murmurs are either tricuspid regurgitation or mitral regurgitation and right-sided murmurs are enhanced on inspiration.

30) b

Diastolic murmurs include: aortic regurgitation, mitral stenosis, pulmonary regurgitation (rare) and tricuspid stenosis (rare). The presence of an S3 heart sound and location are suggestive of aortic regurgitation.

31) f

The ALS algorithm for tachycardia advocates amiodarone 300mg IV over 20-60 minutes, then 900mg over 24 hours.

32) c

The ALS algorithm for tachycardia advocates rate control with beta-blockers or diltiazem for AF.

33) e

The ALS algorithm for tachycardia advocates initial vagal manoeuvres for a regular narrow complex tachycardia.

34)  d

The ALS algorithm for tachycardia advocates initial vagal manoeuvres for a regular narrow complex tachycardia and if this fails, commence 6mg adenosine by a rapid IV bolus.

35)  g

Polymorphic tachycardia is associated with long QT syndrome and is treated using intravenous magnesium.

36)  b

Glucagon is the treatment for beta-blocker overdose.

37)  e

Transvenous pacing may be required if transcutaneous pacing fails to reverse bradycardia.

38)  g

The ALS algorithm for bradycardia advocates observations of a stable patient who has no risk of asystole.

39)  a

The ALS algorithm for bradycardia advocates atropine for a bradycardic patient with adverse features such as syncope.

40)  d

The ALS algorithm for bradycardia advocates transcutaneous pacing if a bradycardia is not reversed following atropine.

41)  g

This is an arrhythmia causing a prolonged QT interval. It may present as ventricular fibrillation, syncope, torsade de pointes or ear abnormalities. It may be treated with a left stellate ganglion block which is a temporary measure and if successful in reducing the QT interval, a surgical ganglionectomy may be performed.

42) d

This is characterised by a shortened PR interval with a delta wave.

43) a

This is characterised by sudden cardiac death and a coved ST segment on ECG.

44) f

This is a long QT syndrome associated with profound bilateral sensorineural hearing loss.

45) e

This is characterised by a shortened PR interval without a delta wave.

# Short answer question answers

1)

a. Any 2 from: 2 marks
- Pericardial rub on auscultation.
- Quiet heart sounds.
- Raised JVP if there is an associated pericardial effusion.

b. Any 1 from: 1 mark
- ST elevation.
- PR depression.

c. Any 4 from: 4 marks
- Infective: viral, bacterial, atypical bacteria, fungi.
- Malignancy (especially lymphoma).
- Uraemia.
- Complication of myocardial infarction.
- Drugs: penicillin, procainamide, hydralazine, isoniazid.
- Autoimmune: SLE, radiotherapy, rheumatoid arthritis.

d. NSAIDs and colchicine. 2 marks

e. A transthoracic echocardiogram to rule out a pericardial effusion and 1 mark
so developing cardiac tamponade.

2)

a. Any 4 from: 4 marks
- Alveolar shadowing.
- Kerly B lines.
- Cardiomegaly.
- Upper lobe diversion (bat winging).
- Blunting of costophrenic angles.
- Fluid in fissures.

b. Any 3 from:                                                    3 marks
- Ischaemic heart disease.
- Dilated cardiomyopathy.
- Hypertensive cardiomyopathy.
- Aortic or mitral valve disease.

c. Any 1 from:                                                    1 mark
- Intravenous furosemide.
- Glyceryl trinitrate infusion.

d. New York Heart Association Classification.                     1 mark

e. Any 1 from:                                                    1 mark
- Cardiac: arrhythmia, MI, acute myocarditis.
- Renal: renal artery stenosis, ACE inhibitor reaction.
- Sepsis.
- Excessive fluid intake.

3)

a. *Staphylococcus aureus*.                                       1 mark

b. Tricuspid valve.                                               1 mark

c. Duke criteria.                                                 1 mark

d. Any 4 from:                                                    4 marks
- Prosthetic valves.
- Intravenous drug use.
- Dental caries.
- Degenerative valvular disease.
- Immunosuppression.
- Rheumatic fever.
- Structural heart disease.

e. Blood cultures.                                                3 marks
ECG.
Echocardiogram.

4)

a. Any 4 from:  4 marks
- Loading with aspirin and one other antiplatelet agent (typically ticagrelor or clopidogrel).
- Nitrates (glyceryl trinitrate sublingual or infusion).
- Diamorphine.

b. Any 1 from:  1 mark
- Percutaneous coronary intervention.
- Thrombolysis.

c. Left anterior descending coronary artery.  1 mark

d. >94%.  1 mark

e. Any 3 from:  3 marks
- Pericarditis.
- Rupture (myomalacia cordis).
- Tamponade.
- Mitral regurgitation.
- Septal defects.
- Arrhythmias.
- Ventricular failure.
- Embolism.
- Dressler's syndrome.
- Death.

5)

a. Any 4 from:  4 marks
- Irregularly irregular pulse.
- Elevated JVP.
- Displaced apex beat.
- S3 (gallop) rhythm.
- Peripheral oedema.
- Bi-basal crepitations.
- Dullness to percussion bi-basally.
- Reduced vocal fremitus bi-basally.
- Murmurs (most commonly functional mitral regurgitation).

b.   ECG.                                                   3 marks

      CXR.

      Transthoracic echocardiogram.

c.   Tachyarrhythmia.                                  1 mark

d.   Dilated cardiomyopathy.                      1 mark

e.   Bed rest until cardiac function significantly improves.    1 mark

6)

a.   An angiotensin-converting enzyme inhibitor (e.g. ramipril).   1 mark

b.   Any 4 from:                                    4 marks

- Cardiac (ischaemia, left ventricular hypertrophy, CCF).
- Aortic (aneurysm, dissection).
- Neurology (cerebrovascular accident, encephalopathy).
- Hypertensive retinopathy.
- Chronic kidney disease.

c.   Any 2 from:                                    2 marks

- Stop smoking.
- Increase exercise.
- Reduce alcohol intake.
- Reduced salt intake.
- Weight loss (if overweight).

d.   QRISK2.                                        1 mark

e.   Any 2 from:                                    2 marks

- Random glucose.
- HbA1c.
- Lipid profile.
- U&Es.

7)

a.   Any 3 from:                                    3 marks

- Hypertension.
- Diabetes mellitus.

- Obesity.
- Smoking.
- Hypercholesterolaemia.

b.  Any 3 from:                                               3 marks
- Age.
- Gender.
- Family history.
- Genetic (e.g. hyperlipidaemia).

c.  Any 1 from:                                               1 mark
- Chest tightness.
- Heaviness.

d.  Any 2 from:                                               2 marks
- Atorvastatin.
- Aspirin.
- Anti-hypertensives.

e.  Glyceryl trinitrate spray.                               1 mark


8)

a.  Syncope.                                                  3 marks
   Angina.
   Shortness of breath.

b.  Any 2 from:                                               2 marks
- Ejection systolic murmur with radiation to the carotids; this is best heard when the patient is sitting forward.
- At the end of expiration.
- A quiet A2 and S4 can sometimes be heard.

c.  Any 3 from:                                               3 marks
- Quiet/absent A2.
- Left ventricular failure.
- S4.
- Narrow pulse pressure.

d.  Nitrates.                                                 1 mark

e.  Any 1 from:                                                          1 mark

- Valve replacement.
- Balloon valvuloplasty.

Balloon valvuloplasty is used when a patient can't undergo a surgical valve replacement procedure.

9)

a.  Irregularly irregular.                                              1 mark

b.  Absence of P waves.                                                 3 marks
    Narrow complex.
    Irregular.

c.  Any 2 from:                                                         2 marks

- Beta-blockers (e.g. bisoprolol, atenolol, carvedilol, metoprolol).
- Calcium channel blockers (e.g. diltiazem, verapamil).
- Digoxin.

Please note: verapamil or diltiazem should not be prescribed with beta-blockers.

d.  After 48 hours; CHADSVASC score.                                   2 marks

e.  Any 2 from:                                                         2 marks

- Warfarin.
- DOACs (e.g. dabigatran, rivaroxaban, apixaban, edoxaban).

10)

a.  Any 2 from:                                                         2 marks

- Blowing into a syringe.
- Carotid massage.
- Coughing.
- Immersing face into cold water.

b.  Adenosine and beta-blockers.                                       2 marks

c.  Any 1 from:                                                         1 mark

- Cardiac ablation, should the patient be haemodynamically compromised.

- DC cardioversion, should the patient be haemodynamically compromised.

d. Wolff-Parkinson-White syndrome                          2 marks
   Lown-Ganong-Levine syndrome.

e. Any 3 from:                                             3 marks
   - Shock.
   - Syncope.
   - Myocardial ischaemia (suggested by typical chest pain or ischaemic changes on ECG).
   - Heart failure.

## 11)

a. Atropine.                                               1 mark

b. Any 3 from:                                             3 marks
   - Shock.
   - Syncope.
   - Myocardial ischaemia.
   - Heart failure.

c. Any 4 from:                                             4 marks
   - Cardiac: atrioventricular block or sinus disease.
   - Non-cardiac: hypothermia, hyperkalaemia, vasovagal, hypothyroidism.
   - Drug-induced: beta-blockers, diltiazem, verapamil, digoxin, amiodarone.

d. Transcutaneous pacing.                                 1 mark

e. Permanent pacemaker.                                   1 mark

## 12)

a. Group A *Streptococcus*.                               1 mark

b. Jones criteria.                                        1 mark

c. Any 3 from:                                            3 marks
   - Pericarditis.
   - Myocarditis.

- AV block.
- Heart failure.
- Endocarditis.

d.   Any 2 from:                               2 marks
- Benzylpenicillin.
- Aspirin.
- NSAIDs.

e.   Any 3 from:                               3 marks
- Subcutaneous nodules.
- Erythema marginatum.
- Sydenham's chorea.
- Arthritis.

## 13)

a.   Cardiac tamponade.                      2 marks
Thrombus of coronary artery.

b.   Ventricular fibrillation.                 2 marks
Pulseless ventricular tachycardia.

c.   Pulseless electrical activity.            2 marks
Asystole.

d.   30 chest compressions to 2 breaths (30:2).   1 mark

e.   Adrenaline 1:10,000 1mg IV (1 mark) every 3-5 minutes (0.5 marks)  3 marks
and amiodarone 300mg IV (1 mark) after the third shock (0.5 marks).

# Chapter 11

# Respiratory
## ANSWERS

## Single best answers

1) a.
2) d.
3) a.
4) b.
5) d.
6) a.
7) a.
8) d.
9) d.
10) b.
11) d.
12) d.
13) c.
14) b.
15) d.
16) c.
17) b.
18) a.
19) c.
20) a.

21)  c.
22)  c.
23)  b.

# Extended matching question answers

1) h

Of the options, only bronchiectasis is associated with clubbing.

2) c

The signs are suggestive of volume loss on the right side consistent with collapse.

3) e

Contralateral deviation of the trachea and an ipsilateral stony dull percussion is typical of a large pleural effusion.

4) f

Symmetrical hyper-expansion, evidence of a smoking history and bilateral wheeze are typical of emphysema (COPD).

5) d

In contrast to emphysematous changes, chest signs in a pneumothorax are unilateral with hyper-resonance and reduced air entry on the affected side.

6) g

A cough at night and worsening shortness of breath on exercise are typical of asthma. Consideration of environmental triggers is important (e.g. damp living conditions).

7) d

Pleuritic chest pain differentials include: pneumothorax, pericarditis, pleurisy and pulmonary embolism. Given no preceding coryzal or lower respiratory tract symptoms and nothing in the history to suggest venous thromboembolic disease, then a spontaneous pneumothorax is most likely.

8) h

The vignette is suggestive of primary ciliary dyskinesia with subsequent development of bronchiectasis. Cystic fibrosis is rare in ethnic groups other than white Caucasians.

9) b

Upper respiratory tract infections are very common. Rhinorrhoea in the absence of chest signs is strongly suggestive of an upper respiratory tract infection.

10) a

A combination of a productive cough, fever and a history of immunosuppression is indicative of a lower respiratory tract infection.

11) g

This question indicates immunosuppressive therapy for bullous pemphigoid and the higher risk of infection and, therefore, tuberculosis is the most likely diagnosis.

12) d

"Odd nail changes" presumably refers to clubbing. There is no history of recurrent chest infections or previous severe pneumonia. There is no history of heart disease or symptoms of heart failure. Therefore, idiopathic fibrosis is the most likely diagnosis.

13) h

Recurrent chest infections and tuberculosis are both risk factors for developing bronchiectasis.

14) e

A dry cough, weight loss and a change in bowel habit in a 70-year-old male is very suspicious of malignancy. The change in bowel habit is likely secondary to hypercalcaemia or a primary colorectal carcinoma.

15) c

Gradually worsening fatigue and shortness of breath are relatively non-specific symptoms, but the need to be more upright for sleep is typical for heart failure.

16) b

*Staphylococcus aureus* classically follows influenza (although any bacterial infection is more likely).

17) d

The rash is erythema multiforme. In the context of an atypical chest infection, this is a typical presentation of *Mycoplasma*.

18) e

Gastrointestinal signs and an atypical chest infection following a recent holiday is typical for *Legionella*.

19) g

*Chlamydia psittaci* is associated with exposure to captive birds.

20) a

*Streptococcus pneumoniae* remains the most common cause of a bacterial pneumonia.

21) b

Stony dull to percussion is suggestive of a pleural effusion, but there is likely to be an infective process with the recurrence of the fever; hence, an empyema is the most likely diagnosis.

22) c

Clinically, a pleural effusion that resolves with a pneumonia is typical of parapneumonic effusion (in contrast to question 21).

23) h

Abscesses typically produce particularly foul sputum and with a history of intravenous drug use there is an increased risk of septic emboli or atypical presentations of infections.

24) f

Septic shock is defined as evidence of infection with haemodynamic compromise resistant to fluid resuscitation.

25) e

The patient has severe symptoms consistent with sepsis, but there is at least some response to fluid resuscitation; as such, this patient has severe sepsis.

26) b

Bird fancier's lung is caused by exposure to avian proteins in the droppings and feathers of a variety of birds.

27) a

This is caused by exposure to *Aspergillus clavatus* spores.

28) d

This is caused by exposure to *Micropolyspora faeni* inhalation.

29) h

This is caused by exposure to *Thermophilic actinomycetes*.

30) c

This is caused by exposure to *Botrytis*.

31)  a

Adenocarcinomas are the most common lung malignancy in non-smokers and are typically more peripheral.

32)  h

A central lesion in a life-long smoker is suggestive of either a squamous cell carcinoma or small cell carcinoma. The central location of the lesion is highly suggestive of squamous cell carcinoma. The severe constipation is likely due to hypercalcaemia and parathyroid protein which are associated with squamous cell carcinoma.

33)  g

Small cell carcinoma is associated with Cushing's syndrome.

34)  e

Suspect asbestos exposure in individuals that have worked in the construction industry. In the context of a pleural effusion, mesothelioma is extremely likely.

35)  f

Multiple lesions suggest a metastatic process.

36)  d

Superior vena cava obstruction presents as shortness of breath with distention of the neck veins and fluid retention in the arms and face only.

37)  c

Malignancy is a hypercoagulable state and therefore predisposes to venous thromboembolism.

38)  a

Severe, boring pain in a patient with suspected malignancy is highly suspicious of metastases.

39) f

Phrenic nerve palsy is often painless and asymptomatic in patients with limited activity.

40) e

Horner's syndrome is characterised by miosis, ptosis and anhidrosis (the combination of signs depends on the site of the lesion along the sympathetic trunk).

41) c

Bleomycin and busulfan are chemotherapy agents associated with pulmonary fibrosis.

42) e

In a young patient with no other risk factors, pulmonary fibrosis is likely due to a connective tissue disorder/autoimmune condition. In ankylosing spondylitis, lung fibrosis is typically apical. Scleroderma is therefore the most likely diagnosis, because crepitations are audible bi-basally.

43) f

Apical crepitations in a young patient is suggestive of a sero-negative arthropathy.

44) d

Severe upper and midzone fibrosis is typical of coal miner's lung.

45) a

Amiodarone monitoring includes regular spirometry.

# Short answer question answers

## 1)

a. Any 2 from: 2 marks
- Infective: *Mycobacterium, Mycoplasma*.
- Malignancy: lymphoma, carcinoma.
- Interstitial lung disease: extrinsic allergic alveolitis, silicosis.

b. Erythema nodosum. 2 marks

   Lupus pernio.

c. Non-caseating granuloma. 1 mark

d. Any 1 from: 1 mark
- Restrictive pattern.
- Reduced transfer factor.

e. Any four from: 4 marks
- Elevated serum ACE.
- Elevated ESR.
- Elevated calcium.
- Elevated immunoglobulin.
- Deranged LFTs.
- Lymphopenia.

## 2)

a. Any 3 from: 3 marks
- Infections: tuberculosis, leprosy, syphilis, cryptococcus, schistosomiasis.
- Autoimmune: primary biliary cholangitis.
- Vasculitis: giant cell arteritis, granulomatosis with polyangiitis, Takayasu's arteritis, polyarteritis nodosa.

- Interstitial lung disease: extrinsic allergic alveolitis, silicosis.
- Idiopathic: sarcoidosis, Crohn's disease.

b. Rifampicin.     4 marks

   Isoniazid.

   Pyrazinamide.

   Ethambutol.

c. Any 1 from:     1 mark
- Ziehl-Neelsen stain.
- Auramine stain.

d. Any 1 from:     1 mark
- Tuberculin skin test.
- Interferon gamma release assays (e.g. QuantiFERON® Gold and T-spot-TB).

e. Löwenstein-Jensen media.     1 mark

3)

a. Computed tomography pulmonary angiography (CTPA).     1 mark

b. Thrombolysis.     1 mark

c. Any 1 from:     1 mark
- Pulmonary hypertension.
- Right-sided heart failure.

d. Any 4 from:     4 marks
- Gender.
- Pregnancy.
- Malignancy.
- Oral contraceptive pill.
- Hormone replacement therapy.
- Lupus anticoagulant/antiphospholipid antibody.
- Personal or family history of thromboembolism disease.
- Morbid obesity.
- Recent surgery.

- Malignancy.
- Immobility.

e.   Any 3 from: 3 marks
- Sinus tachycardia (most common).
- Right heart strain pattern/T-wave inversion in V1 to V4 (most specific).
- Right bundle branch block.
- S1 Q3 T3 (rare).

4)

a.   Nebulised bronchodilators (salbutamol and ipratropium). 3 marks
Steroids (typically prednisolone 40mg PO).
Doxycycline.

b.   Any 3 from: 3 marks
- IV theophylline.
- Invasive ventilation.
- Non-invasive ventilation.
- Doxapram.

c.   Bronchitis. 2 marks
Emphysema.

d.   Arterial blood gas. 1 mark

e.   Any 1 from: 1 mark
- Bullectomy.
- Lung reduction surgery.

5)

a.   Any 4 from: 4 marks
- PEFR <33%.
- $SpO_2$ <92%.
- Type 2 respiratory failure.
- Silent chest/poor respiratory effort.
- Arrhythmias.

- Cyanosis.
- Hypotension.
- Exhaustion/confusion.

b. Magnesium sulphate.                                      3 marks
   Salbutamol.
   Aminophylline.

c. Any 1 from:                                              1 mark
   - Pneumothorax.
   - Ventilation-induced lung injury.
   - Ventilator-associated pneumonia.

d. Non-rebreathe mask.                                      1 mark

e. Steroids (typically prednisolone 50mg).                 1 mark


6)

a. Any 2 from:                                              2 marks
   - Clubbing.
   - Coarse crepitations.
   - Cyanosis.

b. Any 3 from:                                              2 marks
   - Early in disease: *Staphylococcus aureus, Haemophilus influenzae.*
   - Late in disease: *Pseudomonas aeruginosa, Burkholderia cepacia.*
     *Aspergillus spp.* is also associated with cystic fibrosis but tends to
     have an atypical presentation.

c. Any 2 from:                                              2 marks
   - Sweat test.
   - Genetic screening for common mutations.
   - Faecal elastase.
   - Immunoreactive trypsinogen (in neonates).

d. Any 3 from:                                              3 marks
   - Gastrointestinal: pancreatic insufficiency, cirrhosis, gallstones,
     intestinal obstruction.
   - Endocrine: diabetes mellitus.

- ENT: nasal polyps, sinusitis.
- Miscellaneous: male infertility, osteoporosis, vasculitis.

e.   Autosomal recessive. The most common mutation is ΔF508.          1 mark

**7)**

a.   Blood cultures.                                                  3 marks
     Lactate.
     Monitor urine output.

b.   Give IV antibiotics.                                            3 marks
     High-flow oxygen.
     IV fluids.

c.   Rusty-coloured sputum.                                          1 mark

d.   IV co-amoxiclav.                                                1 mark

e.   Any 2 from:                                                     2 marks
     - Right basal crepitations.
     - Reduced air sounds right base.
     - Increased vocal fremitus right base.

**8)**

a.   Intensive care unit for ventilatory support.                   1 mark

b.   Any 5 from:                                                     5 marks
     - Shock.
     - Sepsis.
     - Multiple transfusions.
     - Major haemhorrhage.
     - Pancreatitis.
     - Disseminated intravascular coagulation.
     - Obstetric disasters.
     - Heroin.
     - Aspirin.
     - Fat embolism.
     - Pneumonia.

- Burns.
- Aspiration.
- Inhalation injury.
- Contusion.
- Near drowning.
- Reperfusion Injury.

c. Bilateral infiltrates.      1 mark

d. Any 2 from:      2 marks
- Ventilation-induced lung injury.
- Ventilation-associated pneumonia.
- Difficulties with weaning from the ventilator.

e. Very poor: 50-75% mortality.      1 mark

9)

a. Any 3 from:      3 marks
- Confusion/drowsiness.
- Headache.
- Flushed appearance.
- Carbon dioxide retention flap.
- Bounding pulse.

b. $PaO_2$ <8kPa.      2 marks
   $PaCO_2$ >6kPa.

c. 88-92%.      1 mark

d. Any 2 from:      2 marks
- Non-invasive ventilation.
- Nasal cannula.
- Venturi mask.

e. Any 2 from:      2 marks
- Clubbing.
- Bi-basal fine inspiratory crepitations.
- Chronic hypoxia.
- Polycythaemia.

- Pulmonary hypertension.
- Loud P2 sound.
- Cor pulmonale.
- Raised JVP.
- Peripheral oedema.

10)

a. Any 3 from: 3 marks
  - Obesity.
  - Male.
  - Smoker.
  - Alcohol excess.
  - Structural airway disease (e.g. micrognathia).
  - Motor neurone disease.
  - Lung fibrosis.

b. Any 3 from: 3 marks
  - Snoring.
  - Apnoeic episodes during sleep.
  - Morning headache.
  - Somnolence.
  - Irritability.
  - Depression.
  - Inattention.
  - Impaired memory.

c. Any 2 from: 2 marks
  - Weight loss.
  - Smoking cessation.
  - Reduce alcohol intake.

d. CPAP at night. 1 mark

e. Any 1 from: 1 mark
  - Tonsillectomy.
  - Uvulopalatopharyngoplasty.

## 11)

a. Any 4 from:      4 marks
- Asthma.
- Allergic bronchopulmonary aspergillosis.
- Aspergilloma.
- Invasive aspergillosis.
- Extrinsic allergic alveolitis.
- Chronic necrotising pulmonary aspergillosis.

b. Itraconazole.      1 mark

c. Bronchiectasis.      1 mark

d. Any 3 from:      3 marks
- Behavioural changes.
- Insomnia.
- Gastritis.
- Gastric ulcers.
- Weight gain.
- Adrenal insufficiency.
- Hypertension.
- Hyperglycaemia.
- Immunosuppression.
- Skin thinning.
- Muscle weakness.

e. Any 1 from:      1 mark
- Elevated eosinophils.
- Elevated immunoglobulin E.

## 12)

a. Any 2 from:      2 marks
- Stoney dull to percussion.
- Reduced air entry on right base.
- Reduced vocal fremitus.
- The trachea may be deviated to the left.
- Reduced air entry on the right.

b.    Dependent homogenous opacification with meniscus.     1 mark

c.    Light's criteria.     1 mark

d.    Any 2 from:     2 marks
- Microscopy and culture of sample.
- Rheumatoid factor.
- Anti-nuclear antibody.
- Complement.
- Cytology.

e.    Any 4 from:     4 marks
- Malignancy.
- Infection.
- Rheumatoid arthritis.
- PE.
- Trauma.
- Rheumatoid arthritis.
- SLE.

13)

a.    Elevate the arms above the head for at least one minute. A positive    1 mark
result would include facial plethora, a raised JVP and inspiratory
stridor.

b.    Face and upper limbs.     1 mark

c.    Any 4 from:     4 marks
- Lung malignancy.
- Thymus malignancy.
- Fibrotic bands.
- Radiotherapy.
- Chemotherapy.
- Lymph nodes.
- Superior vena cava thrombosis.

d.    Lung malignancy.     1 mark

e.    Any 3 from:     3 marks
- Dexamethasone.

- Balloon venoplasty.
- SVC stent.
- Radiotherapy.

# Chapter 12

# Gastroenterology
## ANSWERS

## Single best answers

1)    a.
2)    c.
3)    b.
4)    c.
5)    a.
6)    d.
7)    c.
8)    b.
9)    c.
10)    a.
11)    a.
12)    b.
13)    c.
14)    b.
15)    d.
16)    a.
17)    b.
18)    d.
19)    a.
20)    a.

21) c.
22) b.
23) d.

# Extended matching question answers

1) a

A history of an upper GI bleed combined with a history of alcohol excess and signs of chronic liver failure should indicate oesophageal varices as the cause of this patient's bleeding.

2) d

This patient has an aorto-enteric fistula which is a communication between a repaired aorta and GI tract. It should be considered in any patient who has a history of an open or endovascular repair of an aortic aneurysm. It can result in bloody stools and even death.

3) c

The history of pain worse on eating indicates that the patient has a peptic ulcer; these are divided into duodenal which are relieved with food and gastric which are worsened with food. Treatment involves prescribing proton pump inhibitors or H2 receptor antagonists and addressing the underlying cause such as *H. pylori*, NSAIDs, smoking. Endoscopic intervention is required in bleeding ulcers.

4) b

Severe vomiting leads to a tear in the mucosa at the junction of the stomach and the oesophagus. It is usually a self-limiting condition but may require surgical or endoscopic treatment.

5) h

This is an uncommon cause for an upper GI bleed; however, *H. pylori* is a risk factor for gastric adenocarcinoma. The enlarged hard left supraclavicular lymph node is Troisier's sign indicating a metastatic abdominal malignancy.

6) e

Adenocarcinoma and squamous cell carcinoma are the most common forms of oesophageal malignancy. The progressive history of dysphagia to solids and then liquids indicates an increasing obstruction to the oesophagus and combined with weight loss should point towards malignancy.

7) d

The bird's beak appearance on a barium swallow is characteristic for achalasia which is an oesophageal motility disorder in which there is a failure of the lower oesophageal sphincter to relax and there is a loss of oesophageal peristalsis.

8) f

This patient demonstrates CREST syndrome which is a form of systemic scleroderma; she has Calcinosis, Reynaud's phenomenon, oEsophageal dysmotility, Sclerodactyly and Telangiectasia.

9) c

A hiatus hernia is the prolapse of a portion of the stomach into the thoracic cavity through the oesophageal hiatus located at T10. There are two types of hiatus hernia: sliding and rolling. This case demonstrates a rolling hiatus hernia as a fluid level is not seen in a sliding hernia. Rolling hernias may present with nausea, dysphagia, substernal pain, whilst sliding hiatus hernias present with symptoms of gastro-oesophageal reflux disease (GORD).

10) g

The corkscrew appearance is characteristic of diffuse oesophageal spasm. In this condition, there are uncoordinated contractions of the oesophagus leading to dysphagia and regurgitation. It is usually treated using proton pump inhibitors, calcium channel blockers, nitrates, and some studies have shown endoscopic balloon dilatation or botulinum toxin injected above the lower oesophageal sphincter may provide temporary relief of symptoms.

11)  g

Charcot's triad of jaundice, fever and right upper quadrant pain are the key features of ascending cholangitis. The addition of confusion and hypotension to the other factors of Charcot's triad is known as Reynolds' pentad.

12)  h

Pancreatic cancer is the fifth most common cancer in the UK. It is characterised by epigastric pain radiating to the back, painless jaundice and features of malabsorption. Thrombophlebitis migrans is the transient swelling and redness of different limb veins due to clot formation. It is important to remember Courvoisier's Law in relation to painless jaundice; this states that in the presence of a palpable gallbladder, painless jaundice is unlikely to be due to gallstones. This holds true as the formation of gallstones results in a fibrotic shrunken gallbladder that does not easily distend.

13)  c

Primary sclerosing cholangitis is the progressive fibrosis and inflammation of the intrahepatic and extrahepatic bile ducts; this leads to duct destruction. It is associated with inflammatory bowel disease and HIV. Blood results shows deranged LFTs and positive P-ANCA. A liver biopsy is diagnostic showing polymorph bile duct infiltration. Treatment aims to treat pruritis and minimise episodes of cholangitis. Endoscopic dilatation, stenting or resection may be required.

14)  b

Gilbert's syndrome is an autosomal recessive disorder due to a mutation in the UGT1A1 gene resulting in decreased activity of the UGT enzyme. It is characterised by mild jaundice following fasting, stress or infection. Blood tests will show a raised unconjugated bilirubin. It does not require any treatment.

15) f

Sickle cell anaemia is an autosomal recessive condition in which valine replaces glutamic acid on the p arm of chromosome 11. A sickle cell crisis is a medical emergency as sickle-shaped cells obstruct blood flow leading to a vaso-occlusive crisis. Infection, dehydration and acidosis are triggers. Red blood cells are broken down at a faster rate leading to a rise in unconjugated bilirubin.

16) c

Bacterial gastroenteritis is inflammation of the gastrointestinal tract. Symptoms include diarrhoea and vomiting. The rapid symptom onset indicates a bacterial cause in this case.

17) b

Coeliac disease is an autoimmune disorder from exposure to the α-gliadin portion of gluten. Biopsies will show villous atrophy and crypt hyperplasia. It is a common cause of malabsorption. Coeliac disease mainly affects the proximal small bowel. Clinical features include diarrhoea, steatorrhoea, abdominal pain, bloating, failure to thrive, angular stomatitis and dermatitis herpetiformis which is an itchy vesicular rash commonly affecting the elbows, knees or scalp. Tissue transglutaminase antibodies (tTG) and endomysial antibodies are positive. Treatment involves a lifelong gluten-free diet.

18) d

Whipple's disease is a rare bacterial infection caused by *Tropheryma whipplei*. It is more common in farmers and sewage workers. It usually affects the small bowel. Symptoms include joint pain, steatorrhoea, fever, abdominal pain and lymphadenopathy. Endoscopic biopsies will show the presence of periodic acid-Schiff

(PAS) positive macrophages with intracellular Gram-positive bacilli in the lamina propria. Treatment is with a prolonged antibiotic course for at least 1 year.

19) f

Lactose intolerance is caused by a deficiency in the brush border enzyme, lactase, leading to decreased lactose breakdown and absorption. Symptoms usually occur 1-2 hours after lactose ingestion and include diarrhoea, abdominal bloating, flatulence and borborygmi.

20) g

A carcinoid tumour is a neuroendocrine tumour affecting the gastrointestinal system which produces serotonin (5-HT). It is common at the appendix or terminal ileum but may occur at any point along the GI tract. Symptoms include abdominal pain, GI bleeding, flushing, hypotension and weight loss. Patients can be treated with somatostatin analogues such as octreotide.

21) e

This patient has had an upper GI bleed due to a peptic ulcer which was initially treated using an endoscopic approach. He has experienced a rebleed which is an indication for a partial gastrectomy.

22) c

This patient is presenting with GORD, which is usually treated with a proton pump inhibitor to reduce gastric acid secretion, weight loss and smoking cessation.

23) d

This patient has a positive CLO test indicating *H. pylori* infection, which should be treated with a triple therapy approach of two antibiotics and a proton pump inhibitor. The antibiotic regime used depends on local trust policy. An example is amoxicillin, clarithromycin and omeprazole but many different alternatives can be used.

24) b

This patient is presenting with pernicious anaemia, in which the autoimmune destruction of parietal cells leads to a reduction in intrinsic factor production. It is treated with IM Vitamin $B_{12}$.

25) g

This patient is presenting with Crohn's disease. As this is their first presentation, oral glucocorticoids should be commenced.

26) e

Diverticulitis is the inflammation of outpouchings of the colonic mucosa through a weakened area of the colonic wall (diverticula) with associated abdominal pain, fever and a change in bowel habit.

27) f

The use of broad-spectrum antibiotics leads to a disruption of normal bowel flora leading to overgrowth of *Clostridium difficile* causing diarrhoea and in some cases pseudomembranous colitis. It can be fatal. Treatment is to stop causative antibiotics, fluid support, oral vancomycin and metronidazole.

28) a

Irritable bowel syndrome (IBS) is a chronic disorder characterised by abdominal pain, bloating and a change in bowel habit which occurs in a relapsing-remitting course. The Rome III criteria are used when diagnosing IBS and it is important to exclude red flag symptoms such as unintentional weight loss, rectal bleeding or anaemia prior to establishing an IBS diagnosis.

29) d

Ischaemic colitis is necrosis of a bowel segment due to a reduction in blood supply. The history of ischaemic heart disease is a risk factor. Pain is usually of a sudden onset associated with rectal bleeding. Thumb printing on abdominal X-ray and raised lactate help support the diagnosis.

30) c

Ulcerative colitis generally affects the colon to rectum in a continuous manner. Patients may present with bloody diarrhoea, passage of mucus, abdominal pain, fever, episcleritis, uveitis, scleritis, erythema nodosum or pyoderma gangrenosum.

31) d

Primary biliary cirrhosis is the progressive destruction of intralobular bile ducts leading to cholestasis. It can lead to fibrosis and cirrhosis. It is diagnosed by an elevation in ALP, $\gamma$-GT and positive anti-mitochondrial antibodies.

32) h

Drug-induced liver injury is the dysfunction of the liver due to a causative drug. Many drugs can cause liver damage including isoniazid, amiodarone, alcohol or paracetamol. These drugs can cause hepatitis, cholestasis, steatohepatitis, fibrosis, necrosis or oncogenesis.

33) e

Hepatocellular carcinoma is a malignancy arising from hepatocytes; conditions such as primary sclerosing cholangitis, hepatitis, liver cirrhosis increase the malignancy risk. $\alpha$-fetoprotein will be increased, and symptoms include abdominal pain, jaundice, ascites or signs of chronic liver disease. It can be managed with surgical resection, transplant, chemo-embolisation or systemic chemotherapy.

34) b

Primary sclerosing cholangitis is the progressive fibrosis and inflammation of the intrahepatic and extrahepatic bile ducts. This leads to duct destruction and is associated with inflammatory bowel disease and HIV. Bloods show deranged LFTs and positive P-ANCA. A liver biopsy shows polymorph bile duct infiltration. Treatment aims to treat pruritis and minimise episodes of cholangitis. Endoscopic dilatation, stenting or resection may be required.

35) f

Liver failure is the destruction of hepatocytes resulting in an inability of the liver to perform its essential functions. Symptoms include nausea, fatigue and hepatic encephalopathy due to the failure of the liver to remove nitrogenous compounds from the bloodstream. Asterixis and signs of chronic liver disease such as spider naevi or portal hypertension will be evident.

36) g

Multiple endocrine neoplasia Type 1 is the presence of pituitary tumour, parathyroid hyperplasia and pancreatic tumours. It is caused by a mutation in the MEN1 gene.

37) b

Zollinger-Ellison syndrome is caused by gastrinomas, which are neuroendocrine tumours which secrete gastrin; this leads to multiple peptic ulcers, abdominal pain and diarrhoea. Endoscopy reveals multiple peptic ulcers and a raised fasting serum gastrin.

38) d

Exocrine pancreatic insufficiency is the inability to digest food due to a lack of pancreatic digestive enzymes. It is often found in conditions such as cystic fibrosis and chronic pancreatitis.

39) a

Acute pancreatitis is the inflammation of the pancreas. It is commonly caused by gallstones and alcohol in the UK. The mnemonic 'I GET SMASHED' can be used to remember the causes of pancreatitis. Symptoms include epigastric pain radiating to the back which is severe in nature and is exacerbated by eating, fever or jaundice. Treatment is supportive with fluids, analgesia and maintaining nutrition; nasojejunal feeding is used.

40) c

Pancreatic cancer is the fifth most common cancer in the UK. It is characterised by epigastric pain radiating to the back, painless jaundice and malabsorption. Thrombophlebitis migrans is the transient swelling and redness of different limb veins due to clot formation. It is important to remember Courvoisier's Law in painless jaundice. This holds true as the formation of gallstones results in a fibrotic gallbladder that does not easily distend.

41) g

This patient has autoimmune hepatitis and given the lack of risk factors, such as IV drug use, this makes a diagnosis of hepatitis A-E unlikely. The previous history of an autoimmune condition and positive antibodies lead to the appropriate diagnosis.

42) a

Hepatitis A is transmitted by the faecal-oral route and is often contracted by eating contaminated foods such as shellfish.

43) c

Hepatitis C is common in North Africa and has a similar transmission to Hepatitis B. Symptoms include abdominal pain, joint pain, jaundice and pruritis.

44) d

Hepatitis D infection requires co-infection with hepatitis B; if contracted with acute hepatitis B, a more severe acute hepatitis presentation is seen, whilst infection with chronic hepatitis B causes an acute-on-chronic presentation.

45) f

Long-term alcohol consumption leads to initial steatosis in which fat accumulates in the liver and causes an increase in size. Continued alcohol use leads to inflammation and fibrosis known as steatohepatitis and can progress to scarring and fibrosis (cirrhosis).

# Short answer question answers

1)

a.  Acute liver failure.                                    1 mark

b.  Any 4 from:                                             2 marks
   - Nausea.
   - Vomiting.
   - Diarrhoea.
   - Cholestasis.
   - Fever.
   - Abdominal pain.
   - Fatigue.
   - Anorexia.
   - Coma.
   - Agitation.

c.  Any 4 from:                                             2 marks
   - Asterixis.
   - Hepatomegaly.
   - Splenomegaly.
   - Malaise.
   - Pallor.
   - Ascites.
   - Right upper quadrant pain.
   - Abdominal swelling.

d.  Any 2 from:                                             2 marks
   - Fluid resuscitation.
   - Lactulose.
   - Factor concentrates.
   - Antibiotics.
   - N-acetylcysteine.

- Vitamin K.
- Liver transplantation.

e. Any 3 from:  3 marks
- Hepatorenal syndrome.
- Sepsis.
- Ascites.
- Hypoglycaemia.
- Hepatic encephalopathy.
- Multiple organ failure.
- Coagulopathy.
- Seizures.
- Haemorrhage.
- Acute respiratory distress syndrome (ARDS).

2)

a. Any 4 from:  2 marks
- Obesity.
- Smoking.
- Alcohol.
- Stress.
- Family history.
- Hiatus hernia.
- Gastroparesis.
- High caffeine intake.
- Pregnancy.
- Calcium channel blockers.
- Oestrogen usage.
- Beta-adrenergic agonists.

b. Any 4 from:  2 marks
- Proton pump inhibitor trial.
- Upper GI endoscopy.
- Barium study.

- Oesophageal pH monitoring.
- Oesophageal manometry.
- Gastric emptying studies.

c. Any 4 from:                                                    2 marks

- Dysphagia.
- Odynophagia.
- Weight loss.
- Upper GI bleeding.
- Anaemia.
- Persistent symptoms in those aged >55 years.

d. Any 4 from:                                                    2 marks

- Proton pump inhibitors.
- Antacids.
- H2 receptor blockers.
- Prokinetics.
- Nissen fundoplication.
- Endoscopic gastroplication.
- Endoscopic radio-ablation.

e. Any 4 from:                                                    2 marks

- Barrett's oesophagus.
- Adenocarcinoma.
- Oesophageal stricture.
- Pulmonary fibrosis.
- Chronic cough.
- Asthma.
- Chronic pain.

3)

a. 1 mark for each category and correct example:                 3 marks

- Pre-hepatic: sickle cell, hereditary spherocytosis, pernicious anaemia, thalassaemia, haemolytic disease of the new-born, G6PD deficiency.

- Hepatic: viral hepatitis, autoimmune hepatitis, drug-induced hepatitis, alcohol-induced hepatitis, primary biliary cirrhosis, primary sclerosing cholangitis, Gilbert's syndrome, Crigler-Najjar syndrome, right heart failure, acute Budd-Chiari syndrome, Wilson's disease, non-alcoholic fatty liver disease, leptospirosis, *Cytomegalovirus*, Epstein-Barr virus, hepatocellular carcinoma, decompensated chronic liver disease.
- Post-hepatic: biliary stricture, biliary atresia, gallstones, pancreatitis, primary sclerosing cholangitis, cholangiocarcinoma, carcinoma of the pancreatic head.

b. Plasma bilirubin ≥50μmol/L.    1 mark

c. Pale stools and dark urine.    1 mark

d. Any 4 from:    2 marks
- Viral hepatitis serology.
- Ferritin.
- Transferrin saturation.
- Coeliac screen.
- Caeruloplasmin.
- Immunoglobulins.
- p-ANCA.
- Abdominal ultrasound scan.
- α-fetoprotein.
- Fasting glucose.
- α-1 antitrypsin.
- Anti-smooth muscle antibodies.
- Anti-LKM.
- Anti-nuclear antibodies.
- Anti-mitochondrial antibodies.

e. Any 3 from:    3 marks
- Kernicterus.
- Cholangitis.
- Malabsorption.
- Hepatic or renal failure.
- Hepatocellular carcinoma.
- Cholangiocarcinoma.

4)

a. Tangled cytokeratin intermediate filaments complexed with other   1 mark
proteins such as ubiquitin. They are found in the cytoplasm of
hepatocytes and are associated with alcoholic liver disease, Wilson's
disease and primary biliary cirrhosis (PBC).

b. Long-term damage to the normal liver leads to steatosis in which fat   3 marks
accumulates in the liver and causes an increase in size (1 mark).
Continued damage leads to inflammation and fibrosis known as
steatohepatitis (1 mark). This can progress to scarring and cirrhosis (1
mark).

c. Any 2 from:   2 marks
- Reducing dose of chlordiazepoxide.
- Lorazepam.
- Haloperidol.
- Thiamine.
- Vitamin $B_{12}$.

d. Indicated in chronic liver disease. Patients must usually be abstinent   1 mark
from alcohol for at least 6 months to be considered for
transplantation.

e. Any 3 from:   3 marks
- Steatohepatitis.
- Hepatitis.
- Cirrhosis.
- Addiction.
- Anxiety.
- Depression.
- Portal hypertension.
- Varices.
- Peptic ulcers.
- Pancreatitis.
- Gynaecomastia.
- Spider naevi.
- Ascites.

- Encephalopathy.
- Hepatocellular carcinoma.
- Ataxia.
- Impaired memory.
- Wernicke-Korsakoff syndrome.
- Macrocytic anaemia.
- Cardiomyopathy.
- Chronic gastritis.

5)

a.  Any 4 from:                 4 marks
- IV drug use.
- Contaminated blood products.
- Sexual contact.
- Vertical transmission.
- Breast milk.
- Needle stick injury.

b.  Any 2 from:                 2 marks
- Pegylated interferon-$\alpha$.
- Nucleoside analogues (tenofovir, lamivudine).
- Abstain from alcohol.
- Education regarding sexual contact and drug use.

c.  Any 2 from:                 2 marks
- Cirrhosis.
- Glomerulonephritis.
- Polyarteritis nodosa.
- Fulminant liver failure.
- Hepatocellular carcinoma.

d.  Positive HBsAb, negative anti-HBc, negative HBeAg, negative HBeAb,  1 mark
negative HBsAg.

e.  Hepatitis D.                 1 mark

6)

a.   Any 3 from:                                                3 marks

• Number of stools per day.
• Presence of rectal bleeding.
• Fever.
• Tachycardia.
• Anaemia.
• ESR level.

b.   Any 4 rows from Table 12.1 below.                          4 marks

## Table 12.1

|                          | Ulcerative colitis       | Crohn's disease          |
| ------------------------ | ------------------------ | ------------------------ |
| Age of onset             | 10-30 years              | 10-40 years              |
| Origin                   | Rectum                   | Terminal ileum           |
| Area affected            | Large intestine          | Anywhere along GI tract  |
| Pattern                  | Continuous               | Skip lesions             |
| Thickness of inflammation | Shallow or mucosal      | Transmural               |
| Common symptoms          | Bloody diarrhoea         | Crampy abdominal pain    |
| Diarrhoea                | Common                   | Common                   |
| Malabsorption            | Rare                     | Common                   |
| Complications            | Haemorrhage, toxic megacolon | Fistula, abscess, obstruction |
| Risk of colon cancer     | Marked increase          | Mild increase            |

c.   Any 2 from:                                                1 mark

• Uveitis.
• Episcleritis.
• Conjunctivitis.

- Cirrhosis.
- Chronic hepatitis.
- Renal calculi.
- Ankylosing spondylitis.
- Sacro-ileitis.
- Vasculitis.
- Venous thrombosis.
- Erythema nodosum.
- Pyoderma gangrenosum.

d.  Any 2 from:                                           1 mark
- Colon cancer.
- Toxic megacolon.
- Bowel perforation.
- Primary sclerosing cholangitis.

e.  Any 2 from:                                           1 mark
- Abscess formation.
- Fissures.
- Fistula.
- Skin tags.
- Strictures.
- Obstruction.
- Adhesions.
- Colon cancer.
- Malnutrition.

7)

a.  A-E assessment.                                       1 mark
b.  Any 3 from:                                           3 marks
- Suicide note.
- Planned attempt.
- Staggered overdose.
- Alcohol use.
- Multiple drugs consumed.

- Attempt to conceal suicide.
- Requesting assistance.
- Regret attempt.
- Change in social circumstances.
- Previous suicide attempts.
- Future suicide plan.

c. Any 2 from: 2 marks
- U&Es.
- LFTs.
- Glucose.
- Clotting screen.
- VBG.

d. Paracetamol treatment nomogram. 1 mark

e. Any 3 from: 3 marks
- N-acetylcysteine.
- Oral methionine.
- Activated charcoal if within 1 hour of ingestion.
- Psychiatric review.

8)

a. Irritable bowel syndrome. 1 mark

b. Investigations are usually normal. 1 mark

c. Any 4 from: 4 marks
- Symptom onset ≥6 months prior to diagnosis.
- Recurrent abdominal pain or discomfort for ≥3 days per month for the last 3 months.
- Improvement with defecation.
- Onset associated with change in stool frequency.
- Onset associated with change in stool form.

d. Any 4 from: 2 marks
- Reassurance.
- Physical activity.
- Relaxation.
- Restrict alcohol.

- Regular meals.
- Limit fruit intake to three portions per day.
- Increase fluid intake.
- Low fermentable diet.
- Avoidance of sorbitol-containing foods and drinks.
- Laxatives for constipation.
- Loperamide for diarrhoea.
- Anti-spasmodics, for pain relief.
- Hypnotherapy.
- Cognitive behavioural therapy.

e.  Any 2 from:                                                    2 marks
- Depression.
- Anxiety.
- Stress.

9)

a.  Any 4 from:                                                    4 marks
- *Staphylococcus aureus.*
- *Shigella.*
- *Salmonella.*
- *Campylobacter.*
- *E. coli.*
- *Clostridium difficile.*
- *Yersinia.*
- *Vibrio cholerae.*
- *Bacillus cereus.*
- *Clostridium botulinum.*
- *Clostridium perfringens.*

b.  Any 2 from:                                                    2 marks
- Norovirus.
- Rotavirus.
- Adenovirus.
- Astrovirus.

c.  Any 2 from:                                                          1 mark
    ● Fluid rehydration.
    ● Anti-emetics.
    ● Analgesia.
    ● Electrolyte replacement.

d.  Any 4 from:                                                          2 marks
    ● Patient isolation.
    ● Barrier nursing.
    ● Hand washing.
    ● Personal protective equipment use (gloves, aprons).
    ● Deep clean following patient discharge.
    ● Minimise the number of staff in contact with patient.
    ● Clear signage.
    ● Enforcement of infection control guidelines.

e.  *Clostridium difficile* infection.                                  1 mark


10)

a.  Any 2 from:                                                          1 mark
    ● NSAIDs.
    ● Alcohol.
    ● Smoking.
    ● GORD.
    ● Stress.
    ● *H. pylori.*
    ● Zollinger-Ellison syndrome.
    ● Hiatus hernia.
    ● Oesophagitis.
    ● Spicy food.
    ● Oesophageal spasm.
    ● Oesophageal carcinoma.
    ● Gastritis.
    ● Gastric carcinoma.
    ● Gastroparesis.

- Gallstones.
- Duodenitis.
- Coeliac disease.
- Lactose intolerance.
- Giardiasis.
- Functional disorder.
- Bisphosphonates.
- Aspirin.
- Calcium antagonists.

b. Any 6 from:                                                          3 marks

- Unintentional weight loss.
- Melaena.
- Haematemesis.
- Dysphagia.
- Iron deficiency anaemia.
- Epigastric mass.
- Persistent vomiting.
- Suspicious findings on barium studies.

c. Metaplasia of stratified squamous cells to simple columnar cells.    1 mark

d. Any 3 from:                                                          3 marks

- Endoscopy with a rapid urease test (CLO test).
- Endoscopy + histology.
- Urea breath test.
- *H. pylori* stool antigen.
- Serum *H. pylori* antibody test.

e. Two antibiotics and proton pump inhibitor.                           2 marks


11)

a. Refeeding syndrome.                                                  1 mark

b. Malnutrition Universal Screening Tool (MUST).                        1 mark

c. Any 6 from:                                                          3 marks

- Chronic illness.
- Immunosuppression.

- Chronic pancreatitis.
- Coeliac disease.
- Crohn's disease.
- Alcohol.
- Drug addiction.
- Low income.
- Living alone.
- Malignancy.
- Depression.
- Anorexia nervosa.
- Medications.
- Dysphagia.
- Dementia.
- Mobility issues.
- Dentures.

d. Glucose 4-5g/kg/day.                                                      3 marks
   Protein 0.75g/kg/day.
   Sodium 100-150mmol/day.
   Water 2.5-3L/day.
   Potassium 60-90mmol/day
   Chloride 110mmol/day.

e. Any 2 from:                                                               2 marks
- Treat the underlying cause.
- Nutritional supplements.
- Medications to increase appetite such as prednisolone.
- Mirtazapine.
- Nasogastric (NG) feeding.
- Nasojejunal (NJ) feeding.
- Total parental nutrition (TPN).
- Percutaneous endoscopic gastrostomy (PEG).
- Percutaneous endoscopic jejunostomy (PEJ).
- Surgical gastrostomy.
- Surgical jejunostomy.

## 12)

a.  Any 6 from:          3 marks
- Coeliac disease.
- Ulcerative colitis.
- Crohn's disease.
- Colonic malignancy.
- Laxative abuse.
- Neuroendocrine tumours.
- Bile acid malabsorption.
- HIV.
- Giardiasis.
- Exocrine pancreatic insufficiency.
- Small bowel bacterial overgrowth.
- Tropical sprue.
- Antibiotics.
- Hyperthyroidism.
- Diabetes.
- Addison's disease.
- Hypoparathyroidism.
- Food allergy.
- Small bowel resection.
- Antacids.
- Proton pump inhibitors.

b.  Any 4 from:          2 marks
- Full blood count.
- U&Es.
- Liver function tests.
- Thyroid function tests.
- CRP.
- ESR.
- Glucose.
- Calcium.
- Magnesium.

- Coeliac serology.
- Stool culture.
- Faecal elastase.
- Faecal calprotectin.
- Endoscopy and histology.
- SeHCAT study.

c.  Coeliac disease.                                              1 mark

d.  Any 2 from:                                                   2 marks

- Gluten-free diet.
- Pneumococcal vaccination if hyposplenic.
- Treat nutritional deficiencies.

e.  Any 2 from:                                                   2 marks

- Malabsorption.
- Non-Hodgkin's lymphoma.
- Splenic atrophy.
- Increased risk of GI malignancy.
- Increased risk of other autoimmune conditions.
- Refractory disease.

## 13)

a.  A-E assessment.                                               1 mark

b.  Any 4 from:                                                   2 marks

- Peptic ulcer.
- Oesophagitis.
- Gastritis.
- Duodenitis.
- Oesophageal varices.
- NSAIDs.
- Aspirin.
- Mallory-Weiss tear.
- Upper GI malignancy.
- Angiodysplasia.
- Aorto-enteric fistula.

- Warfarin.
- Corticosteroids.
- Thrombolytic drugs.
- Alcohol.

c. Any 3 from: 3 marks
- Full blood count.
- U&Es.
- Liver function tests.
- Clotting screen.
- Group and save.
- Urgent OGD.
- Terlipressin if there is a suspected variceal bleed.

d. Any 3 from: 3 marks
- Stop any causative medications.
- IV fluids.
- Blood transfusion.
- Major haemorrhage protocol if unstable.
- Urgent OGD with adrenaline.
- Sclerotherapy.
- Variceal banding.
- Argon plasma coagulation.
- Proton pump inhibitor.

e. Blatchford score. 1 mark

# Chapter 13

# Renal
## ANSWERS

Single best answers

1)  a.
2)  c.
3)  d.
4)  c.
5)  d.
6)  d.
7)  c.
8)  b.
9)  b.
10) a.
11) c.
12) a.
13) c.
14) b.
15) a.
16) b.
17) c.
18) c.
19) b.
20) c.

21) b.
22) d.
23) a.

# Extended matching question answers

1) a

The case history shows features of SIRS with a source of infection indicating sepsis. This is a pre-renal cause for acute kidney injury.

2) b

This is inflammation of the renal interstitium. Common causes include infection, or a reaction to a medication such as analgesia or antibiotics. This is a renal cause for acute kidney injury.

3) d

This patient has urinary retention secondary to a blocked catheter. When catheters are *in situ* for long periods, debris can cause a blockage. This is a post-renal cause for acute kidney injury.

4) c

This patient is dehydrated due to a poor oral intake. This is a pre-renal cause for acute kidney injury.

5) d

This patient has a renal stone leading to urinary obstruction. This is a post-renal cause for acute kidney injury.

6) e

Creatinine is a waste product and an increase indicates poor renal function. It is used as a diagnostic indicator to measure the AKI stage.

7) f

Stage 1 is >90ml/min; Stage 2 is 60-89ml/min indicating a mild loss of renal function; Stage 3a is 45-59ml/min indicating a mild to moderate loss of kidney function; Stage 3b is 30-44ml/min indicating a moderate to severe kidney function; Stage 4 is 15-29ml/min indicating a severe loss of kidney function and Stage 5 is <15ml/min indicating kidney failure.

8) h

A normal potassium is usually between 3.5-5.3mmol/L; however, values may vary from hospital to hospital. If raised, the result should be confirmed, an ECG performed and if appropriate hyperkalaemia treatment is given.

9) f

It has been found that race affects GFR. African Americans have a higher GFR than Caucasians and the GFR can be standardised using the Cockcroft-Gault equation which factors in age, race and gender.

10) a

CRP is a useful tool in measuring inflammation; however, it can be raised in several conditions including malignancy and infection. When used in infection it lags behind the WCC.

11) g

Nephrotic syndrome is a classical triad of proteinuria, hypoalbuminaemia and oedema. It is associated with diabetes, glomerulonephritis, amyloidosis, autoimmune conditions and drugs such as gold or penicillamine. Symptoms include weight gain, loss of appetite, nausea, vomiting, frothy urine, hypertension and thrombosis. It is treated using ACE inhibitors, diuretics, anticoagulation and lipid-lowering agents.

12) e

A minimal change disease is glomerulonephritis in which a large amount of protein is present in the urine. It is a cause of nephrotic syndrome. It is known as a minimal change disease as when viewing specimens under a light microscope there are no visible changes but with the invention of electron microscopy, it was discovered the disease is due to a loss of podocyte foot processes.

13)  a

IgA nephropathy is a form of glomerulonephritis caused by the deposition of IgA antibodies in the glomerulus. It is common in young people and the classical presentation is episodic haematuria within a few days of a non-specific upper respiratory tract infection. This is in contrast to post-streptococcal glomerulonephritis which occurs weeks after the initial infection.

14)  f

This is a glomerulonephritis caused by deposition in the glomerular basement membrane and mesangium leading to thickening of both walls. Histopathological findings include proliferation of mesangial and endothelial cells, thickening of peripheral capillary walls and mesangium. The basement membrane is built upon the deposits leading to the tram track appearance.

15)  d

Post-streptococcal glomerulonephritis occurs 10-14 days after an upper respiratory tract infection. It is caused by immune complex deposition within the glomerulus and leads to nephrotic syndrome.

16)  a

Malignancy is an absolute contraindication to organ donation.

17)  f

Chronic rejection develops months to years after transplantation and is caused by alloreactive T and B cells alongside fibrosis of the graft. It is considered irreversible and has a poor response to treatment. A retransplant is normally required.

18) b

Cadaveric donation is the main source of organ transplant. Another form of donation is a live organ donor but this is infrequently used.

19) e

Acute rejection develops days to weeks after transplantation and is a T-cell-mediated immune response against a foreign MHC class. Inflammation and leucocyte infiltration of graft vessels is seen. It is the most common type of transplant rejection and is a Type IV hypersensitivity. It is usually treated with immunosuppression or antibody-based treatments.

20) d

Live organ donation is infrequently used; however, if a matched donor can be found then it may be an option. It is subclassified into whether the organ donor is related to the patient or not.

21) h

The glomerulus is a network of capillaries at the start of a kidney nephron. It receives a blood supply from an afferent arteriole of the renal artery and exits the site via efferent arterioles. The Bowman's capsule and glomerulus are collectively known as the renal corpuscle.

22) g

The distal convoluted tubule is responsible for the regulation of potassium, sodium, calcium and pH via bicarbonate reabsorption and $H^+$ secretion. It is the site of action for aldosterone.

23) e

The thick ascending limb is divided into the medullary and cortical regions. It is impermeable to water. Sodium, potassium and chloride are reabsorbed by active transport. It is a site of action for loop diuretics.

24) d

The collecting duct connects nephrons to a minor calyx and renal pelvis. It is responsible for electrolyte and fluid balance. Aldosterone and antidiuretic hormone (vasopressin) act at this site.

25) h

Diabetic nephropathy is caused by endothelial cell, podocyte and mesangial cell dysfunction producing damage to the glomerular filtration barrier leading to nephrotic syndrome.

26) h

Goodpasture's syndrome is an autoimmune condition in which autoantibodies attack Type IV collagen against glomerular and pulmonary alveolar basement membranes. It causes haematuria, proteinuria, renal failure, pulmonary haemorrhage or haemoptysis. It is diagnosed by renal biopsy and treated with plasmapheresis, steroids, immunosuppression or renal transplantation.

27) c

Blood enters the glomerulus by afferent arterioles and exits via efferent arterioles.

28) f

Renin is produced by the juxtaglomerular apparatus and is released in response to decreased arterial pressure detected by baroreceptors, decreased sodium levels detected by macula densa cells or sympathetic nervous input. It is the first step in the renin-angiotensin-aldosterone system and stimulates the release of angiotensinogen from the liver.

29) e

The macula densa cells are located in the juxtaglomerular apparatus and detect changes in sodium levels to cause the release of renin.

30) b

Blood enters the glomerulus by afferent arterioles and exits via efferent arterioles.

31) b

Erythropoietin is responsible for stimulating red cell production and is released in response to hypoxia. Liver production predominates in the fetal and perinatal period. It is also released by pericytes in the brain.

32) a

Renin is produced by the juxtaglomerular apparatus and is released in response to decreased arterial pressure detected by baroreceptors.

33) d

Angiotensin II is formed from the conversion of angiotensin I by angiotensin-converting enzyme (ACE) and causes vasoconstriction, ADH release and increases aldosterone secretion.

34) f

Calcitriol, which is a form of Vitamin D, is released in response to low levels of calcium and acts to increase uptake of calcium from the gut and increase calcium reabsorption by the kidneys.

35) b

Erythropoietin is responsible for stimulating red cell production and is released in response to hypoxia. Liver production predominates in the fetal and perinatal periods. It is also released by pericytes in the brain.

36) g

Long-term lithium can damage renal cells preventing the ADH response.

37) a

When commencing ACE inhibitors, renal function must be checked to monitor for an acute kidney injury.

38) b

Gentamicin is renally excreted and can cause ototoxicity and nephrotoxicity which is dose-related. It is effective against Gram-negative bacteria and Gram-positive *Staphylococcus*.

39) c

Metformin should be stopped in AKI as 90% is excreted by the kidneys and renal dysfunction will result in accumulation leading to lactic acidosis and an increased risk of hypoglycaemia.

40) f

Trimethoprim is a selective inhibitor of bacterial dihydrofolate reductase preventing tetrahydrofolic acid formation which is utilised in purine formation and subsequent protein, DNA and RNA production.

41) g

Hyaline casts are solidified Tamm-Horsfall mucoprotein that may aggregate in low urinary flow states, concentrated urine or an acidic urinary environment.

42) c

Nephritic syndrome is the presence of haematuria, oliguria, hypertension and glomerulonephritis.

43) e

The presence of white blood cells in the urine should prompt a clinician to assess for a urinary tract infection or other underlying pathology.

44)  b

The most common constituent of a renal stone is calcium oxalate.

45)  f

Waxy casts are suggestive of very low urinary flow and are associated with severe longstanding kidney disease.

# Short answer question answers

## 1)

a. Any 2 from:     2 marks
- Renal artery stenosis.
- Glomerulonephritis.
- CKD.
- Renal malignancy.

b. Autosomal dominant.     2 marks
Autosomal recessive.

c. Any 2 from:     2 marks
- Cysts in liver.
- Berry aneurysm.
- Mitral valve prolapse.
- Male infertility.
- Pancreatic cysts.

d. Systolic >140mmHg.     2 marks
Diastolic >90mmHg.

e. Renal cysts block collecting ducts leading to urinary stasis and stone     2 marks
formation.

## 2)

a. ACE inhibitor.     1 mark

b. Any 2 from:     2 marks
- Anaphylaxis.
- Bronchitis.
- Dyspnoea.
- Muscle cramps.
- Stomatitis.
- Syncope.

c.  Renal artery stenosis.                                          1 mark
d.  Any 4 from:                                                     4 marks
    ● Serum creatinine.
    ● Age.
    ● Gender.
    ● Ethnicity.
e.  Any 2 from:                                                     2 marks
    ● Pregnancy.
    ● Muscle mass.
    ● Eating red meat 12 hours before sample taken.

3)

a.  Renal cell carcinoma.                                           1 mark
b.  Proximal convoluted tubules.                                    1 mark
c.  Any 1 from:                                                     1 mark
    ● Pain.
    ● Palpable mass.
    ● Cachexia.
    ● Pallor.
d.  Any 4 from:                                                     4 marks
    ● Smoking.
    ● Male gender.
    ● Increasing age.
    ● Obesity.
    ● Hypertension.
    ● Family history.
    ● von Hippel-Lindau disease.
e.  Any 3 from:                                                     3 marks
    ● Urinary tract infection.
    ● Benign prostatic hyperplasia.
    ● Acute pyelonephritis.
    ● Alport's syndrome.
    ● Urinary tract stones.
    ● Catheter-related trauma.
    ● Sickle cell anaemia.

- Renal trauma.
- Bladder or urethral trauma.

4)

a. Any 2 from: 4 marks
- Rise in serum creatinine of 26μmol/L or greater within 48 hours.
- 50% or greater increase in serum creatinine.
- A fall in urine output to less than 0.5ml/kg/hour >6 hours.

b. Any 1 from: 1 mark
- NSAIDs.
- ACE inhibitors.
- Angiotensin II receptor blockers.
- Diuretics.
- Aminoglycosides.

c. Any 2 from: 2 marks
- Urine output.
- Fluid balance.
- Blood pressure.
- Heart rate.
- Temperature.

d. Any 2 from: 2 marks
- Sodium.
- Potassium.
- Glucose.
- Creatinine.
- Phosphate.

e. Minimum output = 0.5ml/kg/hour. 0.5 x 75kg x 24 hours=900ml. 1 mark

5)

a. Any 1 from: 1 mark
- 0.9% NaCl.
- Hartmann's solution.

b. Any 4 from:     4 marks
- Refractory pulmonary oedema.
- Persistent hyperkalaemia.
- Acidosis.
- Uraemic encephalopathy.
- Uraemic pericarditis.

c. Stage 4.     1 mark

d. Proteinuria.     1 mark

e. Any 3 from:     3 marks
- Haemodialysis.
- Haemofiltration.
- Peritoneal dialysis.
- Renal transplantation.

6)

a. Any 4 from:     4 marks
- Fatigue.
- Anaemia.
- Anorexia.
- Vomiting.
- Metallic taste.
- Pruritis.
- Restless legs.
- Bone pain.
- Dyspnoea.
- Fluid overload.

b. Any 1 from:     1 mark
- Anhedonia.
- Poor appetite.
- Early waking.
- Psychomotor retardation.
- Reduced ability to concentrate.
- Ideas of worthlessness.
- Recurrent thoughts of suicide.
- Death.

c.  Any 2 from:                                              2 marks
    - Disequilibrium syndrome.
    - Hypotension.
    - Access problems.
    - Thrombosis.
    - Infection.
    - Blockage.
    - Steal syndrome.

d.  Any 2 from:                                              2 marks
    - Peritonitis.
    - Exit site infection.
    - Catheter malfunction.
    - Loss of membrane function.
    - Obesity.
    - Hernias.
    - Back pain.

e.  Any 1 from:                                              1 mark
    - Patient Health Questionnaire-9 (PHQ-9).
    - Hospital Anxiety and Depression Scale (HADS).
    - Beck Depression Inventory (BDI).

7)

a.  Any 3 from:                                              3 marks
    - Tall tented T waves.
    - Flat P waves.
    - Increased PR interval.
    - Ventricular fibrillation.
    - Ventricular tachycardia.
    - Widened QRS complex.

b.  Nebulised salbutamol.                                    3 marks
    Calcium gluconate (10ml of 10%).
    10 units of Actrapid® in 50ml 50% dextrose or insulin.

c.    Any 2 from:           2 marks
- Potassium-sparing diuretics.
- Rhabdomyolysis.
- Metabolic acidosis.
- Iatrogenic.
- Addison's disease.
- Massive blood transfusion.
- Burns.
- ACE inhibitors.
- Artefactual result.

d.    Aldosterone.           1 mark

e.    Adrenal cortex.           1 mark

8)

a.    Urinalysis.           1 mark

b.    Proteinuria.           3 marks
Hypoalbuminaemia.
Oedema.

c.    Minimal change glomerulonephritis.           1 mark

d.    Steroids.           1 mark

e.    Any 4 from:           4 marks
- Membranous nephropathy.
- Thin basement membrane nephropathy.
- Mesangiocapillary glomerulonephritis.
- Focal segmental glomerulosclerosis.
- Membranoproliferative glomerulonephritis.

9)

a.    *E. coli.*           1 mark

b.    Positive nitrites.           2 marks
Evidence of leukocytes.

c.    Trimethoprim — inhibits folic acid synthesis and there is an increased  2 marks
risk of birth defects in the developing foetus before 12 weeks.

d. Urinary tract infection in the presence of an abnormal renal tract.    1 mark

e. Any 4 from:    4 marks
- Catheterisation.
- Outflow obstruction such as calculi or enlarged prostate.
- Sexual intercourse.
- Immunosuppression.
- Pregnancy.
- Diabetes mellitus.
- Recent urological procedures.

## 10)

a. IgA nephropathy.    3 marks

Any 2 from:
- Proteinuria.
- Hypertension.
- Renal failure.

b. IgA immune complexes form.    2 marks

Deposit in mesangial cells.

c. Steroids.    2 marks

Cyclophosphamide.

d. Type III hypersensitivity reaction.    1 mark

e. Any 2 from:    2 marks
- Anti-GBM disease.
- Proliferative glomerulonephritis.
- Rapidly progressive glomerulonephritis.
- Henoch-Schönlein purpura.

## 11)

a. Anti-glomerular basement membrane disease or Goodpasture's syndrome.    1 mark

b. Autoantibodies form (1 mark) to Type IV collagen (1 mark) found in the blood vessel basement membranes within the lungs and kidneys (1 mark).    3 marks

c.   Steroids.                                             3 marks
     Cyclophosphamide.
     Plasma exchange.
d.   Renal biopsy.                                         1 mark
e.   Any 2 from:                                           2 marks
     • Malaise.
     • Weight loss.
     • Arthralgia.
     • Low-grade fever.


12)

a.   Disequilibrium syndrome.                             2 marks
     Rapid changes in plasma osmolality and cerebral oedema.
b.   Any 2 from:                                          2 marks
     • Hypotension.
     • Fistula thrombosis.
     • Stenosis.
     • Aneurysm.
     • Temporary line infection or blockage.
     • Steal syndrome.
c.   Blood flows on one side of a semipermeable membrane (1 mark)   3 marks
     whilst dialysis fluid flows in the opposite direction (1 mark). Solute
     transfer occurs by diffusion (1 mark).
d.   Any 2 from:                                          2 marks
     • Low-salt diet.
     • Moderate protein diet.
     • Calorie controlled diet to maintain healthy weight.
e.   Any 1 from:                                          1 mark
     • Iron deficiency.
     • Decreased renal synthesis of erythropoietin.

13)

a. Rhabdomyolysis. 1 mark

b. Dehydration. 2 marks

AKI secondary to raised CK.

c. Myocardial infarction. 2 marks

ECG.

d. Any 4 from: 4 marks

- Burns.
- Crush injury.
- Excessive exercise.
- Myositis.
- Drugs and toxins: heroin, ecstasy.
- Neurological: neuroleptic malignant syndrome, seizures.
- Infections: Coxsackie, EBV, influenza.
- Electrolytes: low potassium, low phosphate.
- Inherited muscle disorders: Duchenne's muscular dystrophy.

e. IV fluid rehydration. 1 mark

# Chapter 14

# Endocrinology
## ANSWERS

1) b.
2) c.
3) c.
4) a.
5) c.
6) a.
7) b.
8) a.
9) b.
10) b.
11) a.
12) d.
13) c.
14) d.
15) a.
16) d.
17) c.
18) b.
19) a.
20) c.

21) a.
22) b.
23) d.

# Extended matching question answers

1)  f

    Elderly patients who become unwell can have multiple complications, and they often do not eat or drink properly. This can lead to both hyperglycaemia and hypoglycaemia. In this case, given the symptoms, hypoglycaemia secondary to infection is the most likely.

2)  a

    Given the patient's age and symptoms, Type 1 diabetes is likely. There are no typical features of DKA.

3)  g

    Given the history of dementia, confusion over medication, a sudden change in conscious level, an insulin overdose should be suspected.

4)  d

    This is a classical presentation of DKA. This is when lack of insulin leads to fatty acid metabolism and ketone production, causing hyperglycaemia and ketoacidosis.

5)  b

    This history is consistent with a diagnosis of Type 2 diabetes, given the patient's age, the symptoms expressed and increased susceptibility to infections.

6)  b

    Gliclazide is the most common drug to cause hypoglycaemia.

7)  a

    Nausea is the most common side effect of metformin.

8) d

This causes bowel symptoms, including flatulence, as it delays digestion of complex carbohydrates in the intestinal tract.

9) b

Gliclazide causes weight gain and an increased risk of hypoglycaemia.

10) c

DPP-4 inhibitors work by reducing the breakdown of incretins, which increase insulin production. It may cause hepatic dysfunction and pancreatitis.

11) f

The most common cause of hypothyroidism worldwide is iodine deficiency. These symptoms are of hypothyroidism and given the recent location change would make this the most appropriate option.

12) e

These symptoms are consistent with hypothyroidism. The history of Type 1 diabetes signifies an autoimmune history indicating the most likely underlying diagnosis is Hashimoto's thyroiditis.

13) a

These are symptoms of Graves' disease, which is autoimmune hyperthyroidism. Common symptoms and signs include sweating, weight loss and proptosis.

14) g

These are symptoms of hypothyroidism. The recent surgery suggests hypothyroidism secondary to thyroidectomy.

15) d

This presentation is classical of De Quervain's thyroiditis. It is a post-viral thyroiditis causing hyperthyroidism followed by hypothyroidism.

16) a

Peri-oral paraesthesia is a classic feature of low calcium levels. Other symptoms include muscle cramps, tetany and spasms. The symptoms involving the blood pressure cuff is Trousseau's sign. Chvostek's sign is a tapping over the facial nerve producing facial muscle spasm.

17) e

The background of long-term secondary hyperparathyroidism alongside serum markers indicate a diagnosis of tertiary hyperparathyroidism.

18) a

This presentation indicates hypocalcaemia. The ethnicity points towards vitamin D deficiency. Palpitations occur in severe hypocalcaemia.

19) b

This patient is presenting with symptoms of hypercalcaemia. The pain indicates likely renal colic. The cough and smoking history indicate a paraneoplastic cause for symptoms.

20) h

Symptoms of hypocalcaemia with an elevated serum PTH indicates pseudo-hypoparathyroidism.

21) e

Hypertension in a young patient may indicate an endocrine cause for symptoms. Conn's syndrome is caused by an adrenocortical adenoma resulting in primary aldosteronism leading to hypokalaemia.

22) g

The sudden withdrawal of long-term steroids can result in iatrogenic hypoadrenalism referred to as an "Addisonian crisis".

23) b

This patient has features of Cushing's syndrome which has many causes including pituitary adenoma (Cushing's disease) and ectopic ACTH secretion commonly from small cell lung cancers.

24) f

This patient is displaying symptoms of Addison's disease. Muscle wasting, hyperpigmentation and postural hypotension are features of hypoadrenalism.

25) c

This patient has symptoms of Cushing's syndrome which can be caused by long-term steroid use.

26) b

These are symptoms of congenital adrenal hyperplasia (CAH). It is a group of autosomal recessive disorders leading to deficiencies in enzymes involved in steroid synthesis within the adrenal glands. The surgery as a child is likely due to ambiguous genitalia which is often found in female infants with CAH.

27) a

These symptoms are consistent with a phaeochromocytoma. This is a catecholamine-secreting tumour of the adrenal medulla.

28) c

These are features of acromegaly, a disease caused by an excess of growth hormone. This causes bone growth as one feature which causes the limb pain, and appearance changes. The visual changes are caused by a pituitary tumour, which enlarges and compresses the optic chiasm causing a bitemporal hemianopia.

29) e

This patient is presenting with symptoms of hypothyroidism, with no obvious indication of another underlying cause.

30) d

This patient is displaying symptoms of hyperprolactinaemia, which can be caused by drugs (antipsychotics, SSRIs), pathological states (pituitary adenoma of lactotrophs, hypothalamic-pituitary axis dysfunction) or can be physiological (pregnancy and stress).

31) c

This patient's visual symptoms are due to a disturbance at the optic chiasm. The combination of visual changes and hyperthyroidism are likely due to a pituitary tumour of thyrotroph cells producing TSH.

32) f

These symptoms appear generalised and non-specific, but they are of generalised hypopituitarism. These symptoms paired with the recent PPH indicate a pituitary infarction. This is a result of hypovolaemia and reduced circulating volume leading to reduced pituitary perfusion and infarction. This is known as Sheehan's syndrome.

33) b

Acromegaly and headaches imply raised intracranial pressure indicating a pituitary tumour acting as a space-occupying lesion. Somatotrophs are responsible for these symptoms which produce growth hormone.

34) g

The symptoms are of hypopituitarism. The history points towards a previous trauma when a head injury was sustained. Trauma is an important cause of general hypopituitarism.

35) a

The main aspect of the history is of a raised intracranial pressure headache which are red flags. The symptoms of weight gain and a deep voice are consistent with corticosteroid excess.

36) b

Diabetic ketoacidosis is a serious, life-threatening condition which requires prompt management. The pivotal aspects of treatment are IV fluid resuscitation and insulin therapy. It is a lack of insulin which causes a switch from glucose metabolism to fatty acid metabolism producing ketone bodies causing an acidosis and profound dehydration and hypovolaemia.

37) c

This patient is presenting with symptoms of Type 2 diabetes. NICE guidelines recommend metformin as the first medication of choice after lifestyle modification factors have not been successful.

38) e

This patient is having an episode of hypoglycaemia. The management of hypoglycaemia starts with oral glucose if the patient is conscious or IM glucagon if the patient is unconscious.

39) f

Symptomatic hypocalcaemia requires IV correction. Magnesium levels are important as normal magnesium levels are required for normal calcium homeostasis.

40) a

Hypotension not responding to IV fluid resuscitation, associated with recent steroids, raises the possibility of an Addisonian crisis. IV steroids (hydrocortisone) are often required. Common electrolyte abnormalities include hyperkalaemia, hyponatraemia and hyperglycaemia.

41)  h

This patient is showing signs of primary hypoadrenalism (Addison's disease). The biochemical abnormalities support this diagnosis, implying a possible impending Addisonian crisis.

42)  f

This patient is presenting with signs of hypocalcaemia.

43)  a

These symptoms of diabetes include polyuria and polydipsia, lethargy and low energy. The patient's age implies Type 1 diabetes.

44)  e

Polyuria, abdominal pain and lethargy are symptoms of hypercalcaemia. The history of lung cancer with metastases increases this possibility.

45)  d

These are classic symptoms of hypothyroidism.

# Short answer question answers

1)

a.

Any 2 from: 1 mark

- Hyperglycaemia (blood glucose >13.9mmol/L).
- Acidosis.
- Low serum.
- Bicarbonate.
- Positive urine.
- Serum ketones.

b. Any 2 from: 2 marks
- Weight loss.
- Polyuria.
- Polydipsia.
- Headache.

c. Any 3 from: 3 marks
- Dehydration.
- Pear drop breath.
- Kussmaul's breathing.
- Coma.
- Hypotension.

d. Any 2 from: 1 mark
- ECG.
- Mid-stream urine.
- Chest X-ray.
- CT head.

e. Any 3 from: 3 marks
- Crystalloid IV fluid resuscitation.
- Fixed-rate insulin infusion.

- Potassium monitoring and replacement.
- Treating any underlying cause (e.g. infection).

2)

a. Any 2 from:            2 marks
- Vitamin D.
- Parathyroid hormone.
- Phosphate.
- U&Es.
- Serum ACE.

b. Any 3 from:            3 marks
- Bone pains.
- Joint pain.
- Renal stones.
- Psychic groans.
- Confusion.

c. Any 2 from:            2 marks
- Short QTc.
- Osborn (J) waves.
- VF/QRS irregularity.

d. Any 2 from:            2 marks
- Hyperparathyroidism.
- Malignancy.
- TB.
- Sarcoidosis.
- Hyperthyroidism.
- Drug-induced.

e. Any 2 from:            1 mark
- IV fluid.
- IV bisphosphonates.
- Treat the underlying cause.

3)

a.    Any 1 from:                                     1 mark
- Infection.
- Community-acquired pneumonia.
- Lower respiratory tract infection.

b.    Any 3 from:                                    3 marks
- Polydipsia.
- Polyuria.
- Weight loss.
- Weakness.
- Dehydration.
- Coma.

c.    Cerebral oedema.                       2 marks

d.    Any 1 from:                                    2 marks
- Insulin.
- VTE prophylaxis.

e.    Any 1 from:                                    2 marks
- VTE due to hypercoagulable state.
- Stroke.

4)

a.    Goitre.                                              2 marks

b.    Graves' disease.                          2 marks

c.    Any 3 from:                                    3 marks
- Tremor.
- Sweating.
- Palpitations.
- Weakness.
- Weight loss.
- Pruritis.
- Oligomenorrhoea/amenorrhoea.
- Hair loss.
- Muscle wasting.

- Exophthalmos.
- Proptosis.
- Ophthalmoplegia.

d.  Any 2 from: 2 marks
- Beta-blockers.
- Carbimazole.
- Propylthiouracil.
- Radiation.
- Thyroidectomy.

e.  Any 1 from: 1 mark
- AF.
- Congestive cardiac failure.
- Osteoporosis.

5)

a.  Iatrogenic steroids. 2 marks

b.  Any 3 from: 3 marks
- Oedema.
- Weight gain.
- Fatigue.
- Depression.
- Headache.
- Central obesity.
- Easy bruising.
- Deep voice.
- Proximal myopathy.
- Thin shiny skin.
- Purple striae.
- Excess hair.
- Coarse skin.

c.  Any 1 from: 2 marks
- High- or low-dose dexamethasone suppression test.
- Urinary-free cortisol 24h.
- Late night salivary cortisol.

d.  Any 1 from:                                                      2 marks
    ● Imaging — CT chest, abdomen and pelvis.
    ● CXR.
    ● MRI pituitary.
e.  Any 1 from:                                                      1 mark
    ● Osteoporosis.
    ● Infections.
    ● Panhypopituitarism.
    ● Diabetes.
    ● Nelson's syndrome.

6)
a.  Excess aldosterone production from the adrenal cortex.           2 marks
b.  Adrenocortical adenoma.                                          2 marks
c.  CT/MRI of adrenals to check for adenomas or masses.             2 marks
d.  Medical: aldosterone antagonists — spironolactone or eplerenone.  2 marks
    Surgical: resection or adrenalectomy.
e.  Any 2 from:                                                      2 marks
    ● Hypertensive retinopathy.
    ● Hypertensive nephropathy.
    ● MI.
    ● Stroke.

7)
a.  Addison's disease.                                               1 mark
b.  Any 2 from:                                                      2 marks
    ● Hyperpigmentation.
    ● Postural hypotension.
    ● Muscle wasting.
    ● Vitiligo.
c.  Hyponatraemia.                                                   3 marks
    Hyperkalaemia.
    Hypoglycaemia.

d.  Synacthen or ACTH stimulation test.                                    2 marks

e.  Do not stop abruptly.                                                   2 marks

Increase dose in illness.


8)

a.  Any 2 from:                                                            2 marks

- Stress.
- Pregnancy.
- Breast feeding.

b.  Any 3 from:                                                            3 marks

- Reduced/absent menstruation.
- Galactorrhoea.
- Breast tenderness.
- Headaches.
- Reduced libido.
- Sub-fertility.
- Erectile dysfunction.
- Visual defects (bi-temporal hemianopia).

c.  Visual fields.                                                         2 marks

d.  MRI pituitary.                                                         1 mark

e.  Medical: stop offending drugs, e.g. bromocriptine or cabergoline.     2 marks

Surgical: trans-sphenoidal surgery.


9)

a.  Benign pituitary adenoma.                                             2 marks

b.  Any 3 from:                                                           3 marks

- Excess sweating.
- Deep voice.
- Macroglossia.
- Coarse skin.
- Large limbs.
- Frontal bossing.
- Nerve entrapment.
- Goitre.

c. Carpal tunnel syndrome.      2 marks

d. Oral glucose tolerance test.      1 mark

e. Medical: somatostatin analogues, growth hormone receptor    2 marks
antagonists, dopamine agonists.
Surgical: trans-sphenoidal surgery.

**10)**

a. Adrenal medulla.      2 marks

b. Any 1 from:      2 marks
- Multiple endocrine neoplasia (MEN).
- Neurofibromatosis.
- von Hippel-Lindau disease.

c. Any 3 from:      3 marks
- Headache.
- Sweating.
- Palpitations.
- Tremor.
- Nausea.
- Weakness.
- Anxiety.
- Hypertension.
- Postural hypotension.
- Hypertensive retinopathy.
- Fever.

d. Alpha-blockade followed by beta-blockade.      2 marks

e. 10%.      1 mark

**11)**

a. 21 alpha-hydroxylase.      2 marks

b. Any 3 from:      3 marks
- Hirsutism.
- Acne.
- Oligomenorrhoea.

- Subfertility.
- Delayed puberty.
- Salt-wasting form in men — dehydration.
- Vomiting.
- Weight loss.

c.  17-OH progesterone.                                                    2 marks

d.  Glucocorticoid replacement (hydrocortisone).                          2 marks
    Mineralocorticoid replacement (fludrocortisone).

e.  Any 1 from:                                                            1 mark
    - Increase dose of hydrocortisone.
    - May need IV fluid.

## 12)

a.  Failure of the posterior pituitary to produce ADH.                    2 marks

b.  Failure of the kidneys to respond to ADH.                             2 marks

c.  Any 1 from:                                                            1 mark
    - Lithium.
    - Demeclocycline.
    - Colchicine.

d.  Sodium raised.                                                         3 marks
    Plasma osmolarity raised.
    Urine osmolarity low.

e.  Water deprivation test.                                                2 marks

## 13)

a.  Small cell lung cancer.                                                2 marks

b.  Hyponatraemia.                                                         2 marks

c.  Sodium high.                                                           2 marks
    Osmolarity high.

d.  Any 1 from:                                                            1 mark
    - Fluid restriction.
    - Demeclocycline.

e.  Central pontine myelinolysis.                                          3 marks

# Chapter 15

## Neurology
### ANSWERS

## Single best answers

1) d.
2) b.
3) b.
4) c.
5) b.
6) c.
7) c.
8) b.
9) b.
10) c.
11) d.
12) b.
13) a.
14) b.
15) c.
16) b.
17) b.
18) d.
19) c.
20) b.

21)  d.
22)  c.
23)  b.

# Extended matching question answers

1) d

This describes a benign essential tremor, which is usually an intention tremor that is symmetrical and often runs in families.

2) a

This describes hemiballismus, which is caused by damage to the subthalamic nucleus, which is most commonly secondary to a stroke.

3) e

This is typical of early Parkinson's disease. Tremor in Parkinson's disease is usually asymmetrical and can be elicited by distraction.

4) f

This is most likely a simple partial seizure due to the stereotyped movements and normal examination in between. A previous stroke increases the risk of seizures.

5) g

The combination of dysarthria and tremor is suggestive of Wilson's disease. Other clues are the young age of the patient.

6) g

The visual field affected is contralateral to the hemisphere of the brain affected. An inferior quadrantanopia is caused by damage to the superior optic radiations which are found in the parietal lobe.

7) d

A central scotoma can be due to ipsilateral damage to the optic nerve.

8) c

A homonymous left-sided quadrantanopia must be due to a right-sided defect. A superior quadrantanopia will be due to damage to the inferior optic radiations (Meyer's loop) found in the temporal lobe.

9) a

A bitemporal hemianopia is due to damage at the optic chiasm, often due to a pituitary adenoma.

10) f

A complete optic nerve lesion will cause complete monocular visual loss.

11) h

These are all features of a headache due to raised intracranial pressure; therefore, a space-occupying lesion is most likely.

12) d

With an absence of red flag symptoms, this is most likely to be a tension-type headache. This is supported by the pressure-like sensation and the mention of life stressors.

13) b

While the nature of the headache is similar to question 12, the addition of fever and drowsiness raises the suspicion of meningitis.

14) a

There are features of both migraine and tension-type headaches here. However, the frequency of the headaches and continued use of paracetamol and triptans suggest a medication-overuse headache.

15) e

The unilateral nature, photophobia and vomiting are all features of migraine.

16)  c

Wasting and fasciculations are lower motor neurone symptoms, consistent with limb-onset motor neurone disease.

17)  a

The findings of symmetrical upper neurone weakness are consistent with spinal cord compression. The hypercalcaemia points towards bony metastases as a cause.

18)  f

Rapidly progressive ascending weakness with loss of reflexes points to Guillain-Barré syndrome. This is often preceded by sensory changes.

19)  g

Pain, stiffness and malaise in a female of this age is most likely to be due to polymyalgia rheumatica. While there is often a subjective feeling of weakness, power is usually intact.

20)  d

In a female of this age group, a first manifestation of MS is more likely than a stroke, but a stroke would be the next most likely. A diagnosis of MS could not be confirmed, however, until dissemination of lesions in space and time has been demonstrated.

21)  f

This describes a classical generalised tonic-clonic seizure.

22)  d

In an elderly patient, with a history of a fall, a subdural haematoma is most likely. The fall was unwitnessed and therefore a head injury could not have been excluded.

23)  g

Fever, headache and altered mental state are the clinical hallmarks of encephalitis.

24)  a

This describes a typical syncopal episode, precipitated by the hot environment. The quick recovery is typical of a syncopal episode.

25)  h

While this superficially sounds like an epileptic attack, there are features more suggestive of a non-epileptic attack. These include the longer seizure duration, moaning and quick post-ictal recovery.

26)  b

A head injury with a loss of consciousness followed by a lucid period is a typical history of an extradural haemorrhage.

27)  h

The combination of head injury followed by a gradual deterioration is suggestive of a chronic subdural haemorrhage.

28)  a

A sudden-onset headache could be a subarachnoid haemorrhage; however, pregnancy is a prothrombotic state. Seizures frequently occur in cerebral vein thrombosis.

29)  e

This is a classical stroke picture. An irregularly irregular pulse suggests AF as a precipitating cause.

30)  d

This is a typical history of a subarachnoid headache. Meningeal irritation causes neck stiffness.

31)  e

The facial nerve controls the muscles of facial expression and sensation of taste. A VII nerve palsy without forehead sparing suggests a lower motor neurone lesion, i.e. Bell's palsy.

32)  a

A compressive oculomotor nerve lesion (such as one caused by a space-occupying lesion) can cause damage to parasympathetic fibres before the motor fibres; therefore, ptosis and mydriasis occur prior to the development of a down and out position.

33)  c

The history is of trigeminal neuralgia (cranial nerve V).

34)  b

The trochlear nerve innervates the superior oblique muscle and therefore damage causes vertical diplopia. Acute trochlear nerve palsy is most commonly due to head trauma.

35)  d

The abducens nerve controls the movement of the lateral rectus muscle. It is usually the first nerve to be compressed with raised intracranial pressure. Damage causes horizontal diplopia and a failure of lateral gaze (a convergent squint).

36)  f

Brief vacant periods with rapid recovery are typical of childhood absences.

37)  d

This describes a Jacksonian march, a type of focal (or simple partial) seizure.

38) b

The long duration and emotional elements are suggestive of a non-epileptic attack.

39) a

This is a typical presentation of a focal impaired awareness seizure (a complex partial seizure), e.g. of the temporal lobe.

40) c

This is a typical generalised tonic-clonic seizure, with tonic and clonic phases, loss of consciousness and post-ictal drowsiness.

41) d

The history is that of a migraine, for which sumatriptan would be the most appropriate treatment.

42) h

The history and examination are consistent with limb-onset motor neurone disease, for which the only pharmacological treatment is riluzole.

43) a

The history is strongly suggestive of a transient ischaemic attack and therefore 300mg of aspirin should be given.

44) g

The history suggests myasthenia gravis, which often presents with ocular symptoms before becoming generalised. The treatment of myasthenia is with pyridostigmine.

45) e

The history suggests a flare of relapsing-remitting multiple sclerosis, the treatment for which would be methylprednisolone.

# Short answer question answers

1)

a. Lewy body formation. 2 marks

Loss of dopaminergic neurones in the substantia nigra and reduced dopamine in the striatum.

b. Any 1 from: 1 mark
- SNCA.
- LRRK2.
- Parkin.
- PINK1.
- DJ-1.
- GBA.
- VPs35.
- DNAJC6.

c. Any 3 from: 3 marks
- Rigidity.
- Bradykinesia.
- Postural instability.
- Difficulty initiating or stopping movement.
- Micrographia.
- Speech changes.
- Stooping.

d. Any 3 from: 3 marks
- Cognitive impairment.
- Depression.
- Hallucinations.
- Brisk reflex.
- Constipation.
- Sleep disorders.

e.  Any 1 from:                                                    1 mark
    ● Dopamine agonists.
    ● Monoamine-oxidase-B inhibitors.
    ● Anticholinergics.
    ● Catechol-O-methyltransferase inhibitors.

2)

a.  Any 2 from:                                                    2 marks
    ● Hypertension.
    ● Smoking.
    ● Diabetes.
    ● Valvular heart disease.
    ● Ischaemic heart disease.
    ● AF.
    ● Peripheral arterial disease.
    ● Polycythaemia rubra vera.
    ● Carotid artery occlusion.
    ● Combined oral contraceptive pill.
    ● Hypercholesterolaemia.
    ● Alcohol excess.
    ● Coagulopathies.

b.  CT or MRI head.                                                4 marks
    Echocardiography.
    24-hour ECG (for AF).
    Carotid Doppler (stenosis ≥70%).

c.  5; he scores 1 point for age, 1 for blood pressure, 2 for clinical features   1 mark
    and 1 for duration of symptoms.

d.  300mg aspirin.                                                 2 marks

e.  As an HGV driver, his license will be revoked for 1 year.     1 mark

3)

a. Any 2 from: 2 marks
- Jaw claudication.
- Visual disturbance (e.g. blurred vision, amaurosis fugax, transient or permanent loss, diplopia).
- Anorexia.
- Weight loss.
- Fever.
- Sweats.
- Palpable temporal artery.
- Carotid bruits.
- Muscle/joint tenderness.

b. Temporal artery biopsy. 1 mark

c. Any 4 from: 4 marks
- Cataract.
- Diabetes.
- Immune suppression.
- Osteoporosis.
- Striae.
- Adrenal suppression.
- Peptic ulcers.
- Candidiasis.
- Pancreatitis.
- Skin thinning.
- Hirsutism.
- Bruising.
- Increased sweating.
- Acne.
- Impaired wound healing.
- Raised white cells.
- Weight gain.
- Menstrual irregularities.
- Myopathy.

- Behavioural changes.
- Hypertension.
- Elevated cholesterol.
- Fluid retention.

d. Any 2 from:     2 marks
- Visual loss.
- Aortic aneurysm or dissection.
- Stenotic lesions of major vessels.
- Seizures.
- Stroke.

e. Polymyalgia rheumatica, occurs in 50% of patients.     1 mark

4)

a. Autosomal dominant.     1 mark

b. Chromosome 4.     1 mark

c. Expansion of CAG triplet repeats (1 mark) in the huntingtin gene (1 mark).     2 marks

d. Any 3 from:     3 marks
- Personality change.
- Self-neglect.
- Apathy.
- Depression.
- Dementia/cognitive impairment.
- Irritability.
- Dysphoria.
- Agitation.
- Anxiety.
- Poor judgement.
- Inflexibility.
- Aggression.

e. Any 3 from:     3 marks
- Rigidity.
- Seizures.
- Dysarthria.

- Parkinsonism.
- Dystonia.
- Dysphagia.
- Supranuclear gaze palsy.
- Tics.
- Clonus.
- Bradykinesia.
- Spasticity.
- Extensor plantars.

5)

a. Any 3 from:                                                    3 marks

- Vascular dementia.
- Lewy body dementia.
- Fronto-temporal dementia.
- AIDS dementia complex.
- Korsakoff's syndrome.
- Huntington's disease.
- Hypothyroidism.
- $B_{12}$ deficiency.
- Folate deficiency.
- Neurosyphilis.
- Pellagra.
- Space-occupying lesions.
- Normal pressure hydrocephalus.
- Delirium.
- Schizophrenia.
- Depression.

b. Apolipoprotein E4 variant.         1 mark

c. Amyloid accumulates in senile plaques and hyperphosphorylated tau  2 marks
protein accumulates as neurofibrillary tangles (1 mark) resulting in
neuronal loss and atrophy with subsequent reduction in acetylcholine
(1 mark).

d.  Any 2 from:                                                        2 marks
    - Difficulty with word finding.
    - Forgetting appointments.
    - Difficulty with language.
    - Apraxia.
    - Problems with planning and decision making.
    - Confusion.
    - Wandering.
    - Disorientation.
    - Apathy.
    - Depression.
    - Hallucinations.
    - Delusions.
    - Disinhibition.
    - Aggression.
    - Agitation.
    - Altered eating habits.
    - Incontinence.

e.  Cholinesterase inhibitors (e.g. donepezil, galantamine).          2 marks
    NMDA receptor partial antagonists (memantine).

6)

a.  Any 2 from:                                                        2 marks
    - Superoxide dismutase-1 (SOD1).
    - TARDBP.
    - FUS.
    - C9ORF72.

b.  Any 3 from:                                                        3 marks
    - Wasting.
    - Fasciculation.
    - Absent or reduced reflexes.
    - Reduced tone.

c.  Any 3 from:                                        3 marks
    - Increased tone.
    - Brisk reflexes.
    - Up-going plantars.
    - Clonus.
d.  Non-invasive ventilation.                          1 mark
e.  Riluzole.                                          1 mark

7)
a.  Any 2 from:                                        2 marks
    - Trauma.
    - Vertebral fracture.
    - Tumours.
    - Prolapsed intervertebral disc.
    - Epidural haematoma.
    - Subdural haematoma.
    - Rheumatoid arthritis.
    - Spinal infection.
    - Degenerative spinal disease.
b.  MRI spine.                                         1 mark
c.  Spinal surgery is the only definitive treatment.   1 mark
d.  Any 3 from:                                        3 marks
    - Dexamethasone.
    - Radiotherapy.
    - Analgesia.
    - Bisphosphonates.
e.  Any 3 from:                                        3 marks
    - Pressure sores.
    - Hypothermia.
    - Aspiration.
    - Pneumonia.
    - Acute respiratory distress syndrome.
    - Depression.

- Autonomic dysfunction.
- Sphincter disturbance.

8)

a. Left middle cerebral artery.      1 mark

b. 4.5 hours.      1 mark

c. Any 4 from:      4 marks
- Seizure at onset of stroke.
- Symptoms suggestive of subarachnoid haemorrhage.
- Stroke or serious head injury within last 3 months.
- Major surgery or serious trauma within 2 weeks.
- Previous intracranial haemorrhage.
- Intracranial neoplasm.
- Arteriovenous malformation (AVM).
- Aneurysm.
- Gastrointestinal or urinary tract haemorrhage within the last 3 weeks.
- Lumbar puncture in the preceding week.
- Current anticoagulation with an INR >1.7.
- Acute pericarditis.

d. Aspirin 300mg.      1 mark

e. Any 3 from:      3 marks
- Clopidogrel (P2Y12 receptor inhibitor).
- Aspirin (salicylate).
- Dipyridamole (phosphodiesterase inhibitors).
- Warfarin.
- Direct-acting oral anticoagulants (DOAC), e.g. rivaroxaban.
- Statins (HMG-CoA reductase inhibitor).
- Calcium channel blockers.
- ACE inhibitors.
- Angiotensin receptor blockers.
- Thiazide diuretics.

9)

a. Any 4 from: 4 marks
- Full blood count.
- Glucose.
- U&Es.
- Calcium.
- Magnesium.
- Liver function.
- Coagulation.

b. Advise that she cannot drive home and that she needs to inform the DVLA. 2 marks

She will not be able to drive for at least 6 months.

c. Absence seizure. 1 mark

d. Electroencephalogram (EEG). 2 marks

3Hz spike and wave pattern.

e. Any 1 from: 1 mark
- Ethosuximide.
- Sodium valproate.

10)

a. Any 4 from: 4 marks
- Fatigable muscle weakness.
- Proximal muscle weakness.
- Difficulty getting out of chairs or brushing hair.
- Slurred speech.
- Drooping jaw.
- Difficulty chewing.
- Head droop.
- Issues with anaesthetics (suxamethonium resistance).
- Respiratory failure.
- Fatigable reflexes.

b. Any 2 from:                                 2 marks
- Anti-MuSK.
- Anti-acetylcholine receptor.
- Anti-LRP4.

c. Any 1 from:                                    1 mark
- Tensilon (edrophonium) test.
- Ice test (improvement of ptosis when crushed ice in a latex glove is placed over the eye).
- Repetitive nerve stimulation.
- Mediastinal imaging.

d. Any 2 from:                                 2 marks
- Pyridostigmine.
- Corticosteroids.
- Analgesia.

e. Thymectomy.                                   1 mark

11)

a. Saccular (berry) aneurysm.                      1 mark

b. Xanthochromia (1 mark) on lumbar puncture (1 mark).    2 marks

c. Cerebral angiography.                            2 marks
CT angiography.

d. Sentinel bleeds which are small leaks from the aneurysm.   1 mark

e. Any 2 from:                                   4 marks
- Rebleeding is prevented by occluding the aneurysm.
- Vasospasm is prevented by calcium channel antagonists.
- Hydrocephalus. This is treated by lumbar puncture or ventricular drainage depending on the site of obstruction.
- Pain is treated with analgesia.
- Vomiting can be treated with antiemetics.

## 12)

a. A CT is often performed to rule out raised intracranial pressure as this   1 mark
would increase the risk of uncal or tonsillar herniation.

b. Any 3 from:   3 marks
- Turbid fluid.
- Raised polymorphs.
- Raised protein.
- Low glucose.

c. Any 2 from:   2 marks
- *Streptococcus pneumoniae*.
- *Haemophilus influenzae* type b.
- *Neisseria meningitidis*.
- *Listeria monocytogenes*.

d. Intravenous cephalosporin antibiotic.   1 mark

e. Any 2 from:   3 marks
- Sepsis.
- DIC.
- Coma.
- Cerebral oedema.
- Septic arthritis.
- Pericardial effusion.
- Haemolytic anaemia.
- SIADH.
- Seizures.

Any 1 from:
- Hearing loss.
- Cranial nerve dysfunction.
- Seizures.
- Focal paralysis.
- Subdural effusions.
- Hydrocephalus.
- Intellectual deficits.
- Ataxia.

- Blindness,
- Waterhouse-Friderichsen syndrome.
- Peripheral gangrene.

13)

a. Any 2 from:                                          2 marks
- Worse on waking.
- Postural.
- Worse on coughing.

b. Left abducens nerve.                                 1 mark

c. Any 4 from:                                          4 marks
- Nausea and vomiting.
- Papilloedema.
- Ataxia.
- Seizures.
- Reduced consciousness.
- Focal neurology.

d. CT or MRI of the head.                               1 mark

e. Any 2 from:                                          2 marks
- Surgical resection.
- Radiotherapy.
- Chemotherapy.

# Chapter 16

# Haematology
## ANSWERS

## Single best answers

1) a.
2) d.
3) d.
4) c.
5) d.
6) d.
7) b.
8) d.
9) a.
10) b.
11) a.
12) c.
13) b.
14) d.
15) d.
16) b.
17) a.
18) b.
19) d.
20) a.

21)  c.
22)  d.
23)  d.

# Extended matching question answers

1)　e

Pencil cells can be seen in patients with iron deficiency anaemia.

2)　c

Heinz bodies can be seen in patient with G6PD deficiency; typically these patients can have a haemolytic response when fava beans are ingested.

3)　h

Smear cells are pathognomonic of chronic lymphocytic leukaemia.

4)　b

Helmet cells are seen in patients with microangiopathic haemolytic anaemia.

5)　a

Teardrop cells are pathognomonic of myelofibrosis. The history of fatigue, splenomegaly and weight loss is typical.

6)　a

Down's syndrome is strongly associated with the development of leukaemia — particularly acute lymphoblastic leukaemia.

7)　b

Polycythaemia rubra vera (PRV) is associated with progression to chronic myeloid leukaemia.

8)  f

SLE is strongly associated with idiopathic thrombocytopenic purpura (ITP). Other associations include autoimmune haemolytic anaemia, viral infections and antiphospholipid syndromes.

9)  c

Long-term immunosuppression is associated with the development of non-Hodgkin's lymphoma.

10)  g

Haemophilia is an X-Linked condition and often runs in families.

11)  c

The Ann Arbor staging is used to stage Hodgkin's lymphoma. Stage 3 has lymph nodes on both sides of the diaphragm.

12)  e

Stage 1B describes one region of involved lymph nodes, with B symptoms (unexplained weight loss, recurrent fever, recurrent night sweats).

13)  h

Stage 4B shows diffuse involvement of one or more extra-lymphatic organs with the presence of B symptoms.

14)  a

A single lymph node involvement with no B symptoms.

15)  a

A single lymphatic system affected with no B symptoms.

16) f

Factor XII activates the intrinsic pathway by binding to exposed/damaged collagen. Deficiency of factor XII results in a pro-thrombotic state.

17) d

Factor IX is deficient in Christmas disease (haemophilia B).

18) e

Factor Xa is inhibited by these drugs, resulting in an anticoagulant state.

19) a

Tissue factor (factor III) is an integral part of the extrinsic pathway; it activates factor X to Xa.

20) g

Factor XIII stabilises the fibrin molecules with cross-links; it ensures clot longevity.

21) b

Heparin inhibits factor Xa, thus resulting in an anticoagulant effect. Heparin infusions are usually monitored and titrated using the APTT ratios.

22) f

Warfarin is monitored using the INR. This is calculated by standardising the prothrombin time. Warfarin inhibits factors II, VII, IX and X which are part of the extrinsic pathways.

23) c

Factor II would result in an elevated APTT and PT as it links both the intrinsic and extrinsic pathway.

24) a

DIC occurs due to consumption of clotting factors in the blood. Patients also develop thrombocytopenia. D-dimer levels will be raised as it is a degradation product.

25) d

Patients with von Willebrand's disease have a normal clotting screen and normal platelet levels. Those with von Willebrand's disease often bruise and bleed easily.

26) a

Alpha thalassaemia major is incompatible with life, resulting in hydrops fetalis.

27) d

Sickle cell disease is as a result of an adenine for thymine substitution. Valine is hydrophobic so the haemoglobin molecules 'sickle' particularly when exposed to stress.

28) g

Factor V Leiden is the commonest prothrombotic condition. When this is deficient it cannot bind factor V, resulting in a prothrombotic state.

29) e

G6PD deficiency is most commonly seen in Mediterranean individuals. It causes neonatal jaundice due to haemolysis.

30) b

Beta thalassaemia is more common in Mediterranean individuals. It is treated with blood transfusions to prevent symptomatic anaemia and desferrioxamine is used to prevent iron overload.

31) b

Basophilic stippling is a common finding in patients with beta thalassaemia.

32) d

Sickle cells can be seen on the blood films of patients with sickle cell disease.

33) a

Howell-Jolly bodies can be seen when patients have had a splenectomy. Howell-Jolly bodies contain nuclear remnants.

34) e

Fragmented cells can be seen in patients who have mechanical heart valves.

35) g

Teardrop cells are pathognomonic of patients with myelofibrosis.

36) b

T-helper cells have CD4+ glycoprotein expressed on their surface.

37) a

Neutrophils are typically multi-lobed; they ingest bacteria and damaged tissues. They compose approximately 60% of our circulating white cells.

38) h

Eosinophils produce histamine and have a bilobed nucleus.

39) e

A normoblast is the precursor to a reticulocyte. Reticulocytes are immature red blood cells.

40) f

Megakaryocytes are giant multi-nucleated cells. Once they are fully mature they develop into hundreds of platelets.

41) h

Warm autoimmune haemolytic anaemia is strongly associated with other autoimmune conditions such as lupus. The jaundice shows the patient is 'haemolysing' and blood test results would reflect this.

42) g

March haemoglobinuria describes haemolysis secondary to a 'mechanical' process such as marathon running.

43) d

Red blood cells are more rigid due to the lack of ATP production and are haemolysed. Blood films show poikilocytes and prickle cells.

44) c

Haemolysis is triggered by oxidative stress, infections and fava beans. A G6PD deficiency is most common in the Mediterranean population.

45) a

In hereditary spherocytosis, there is a protein deficiency resulting in a progressive loss of membrane structure and a change in the shape of red blood cells. These spherocytes are prone to haemolysis.

# Short answer question answers

1)
a. Any 3 from:                                                    3 marks
   - U&Es.
   - Urinary testing for light chains (Bence Jones protein).
   - Serum electrophoresis.
   - Bone marrow aspiration.
b. Light chains present in the urine.                             1 mark
c. Clonal proliferation of plasma cells.                         2 marks
   Paraprotein production.
d. Monoclonal gammopathy of undetermined significance (MGUS).    2 marks
e. Any 2 from:                                                    2 marks
   - Chemotherapy.
   - Allogenic stem cells.
   - Bisphosphonate.

2)
a. Chronic myeloid leukaemia.                                    1 mark
b. t(9:22.)                                                       2 marks
c. BCR/ABL.                                                       1 mark
d. Imatinib.                                                      4 marks
   Tyrosine kinase inhibitor.
e. Acute myelogenous leukaemia (AML) or acute lymphoblastic      2 marks
   leukaemia (ALL). Worse prognosis.

3)
a. Any 4 from:                                                    4 marks
   - Hypertension.
   - Abnormal renal function.

- Abnormal liver function.
- Stroke.
- Bleeding.
- Labile INR.
- Elderly.
- Alcohol/drug abuse.

b.  INR 2.5.                                             1 mark

c.  Intravenous vitamin K.                              1 mark

d.  Prothrombin complex concentrate.                    1 mark

e.  Any 3 from:                                         3 marks

- Co-trimoxazole.
- Isoniazid.
- Macrolides.
- Metronidazole.
- Quinolones.
- Tetracyclines.

4)

a.  Ultrasound-guided biopsy.                           1 mark

b.  Ann Arbor staging.                                  1 mark

c.  Any 3 from:                                         5 marks

- B symptoms: fever, weight loss >10% in 6 months, night sweats.

Any 2 from:

- Other symptoms: itching, alcohol-induced pain, back pain, easy bruising.

d.  Reed Sternberg cell.                                1 mark

e.  LDH.                                                2 marks

5)

a.  Autosomal recessive.                                1 mark

b.  Sickling results in vessel occlusion (1 mark).      3 marks

Any 2 from:

- Hyperaemia.

- Infection.
- Dehydration.

c. Any 2 from:     2 marks
- Dactylitis.
- Splenic sequestration crisis.
- Splenic infarction.
- Priapism.
- Aplastic crisis.

d. Transformation to adult haemoglobin complete.     2 marks
Fetal Hb protective against sickling.

e. Bone marrow infarction.     2 marks
Treated with IV fluids.

6)

a. Any 4 from:     2 marks
- Breathlessness.
- Haemoptysis.
- Chest pain.
- Blackout.
- Palpitations.

b. PERC score.     3 marks
Wells score.
D-dimer.

c. Sinus tachycardia.     1 mark

d. Any 4 from:     2 marks
- Chest X-ray.
- Blood tests.
- Urine dip.
- CT of the chest, abdomen and pelvis.
- Mammogram.

e. 6 months.     2 marks

7)

a. A-E assessment. 2 marks

b. O negative. 2 marks

c. O+ (0.5 marks), O- (0.5 marks), A+ (0.5 marks), A- (0.5 marks). 2 marks

d. Any 2 from: 2 marks
- Infections (BBV [rare], bacterial, CJD).
- Transfusion-related acute lung injury.
- Allergic reaction.
- Mismatched blood.
- Circulatory overload.
- Air embolism.
- Thrombophlebitis.
- Hypothermia.

e. Any 2 from: 2 marks
- Cryoprecipitate: factor VIII, VWF, fibrinogen, factor XIII.
- Plasma: contains all clotting factors.

8)

a. Any 3 from: 3 marks
- Diffuse thrombin activation by a trigger.
- Coagulation cascade activation.
- Platelet consumption.
- Clotting factors consumption, leading to disseminated intravascular coagulation.

b. Any 1 from: 1 mark
- Elevated PT.
- Elevated APTT.
- Elevated D-dimer.
- Decreased fibrinogen.
- Decreased platelets.

c. Any 2 from: 2 marks
- Sepsis.
- Trauma.

- Malignancy.
- Placental abruption.
- Amniotic fluid embolism.
- Retained fetus.
- Uterine atony.
- Vasculitis.
- Liver disease.
- Toxins.
- Fat embolism.
- Pancreatitis.

d.   Increased fibrinogen breakdown.                          2 marks
     D-dimer is a fibrinogen degradation product.

e.   Fragmented cells.                                        2 marks
     Thrombocytopenia.


9)

a.   Mutation affecting the ability to produce beta chains (1 mark). Beta   2 marks
     thalassaemia major = homozygous mutation, beta thalassaemia trait
     = heterozygous mutation (1 mark).

b.   Any 3 from:                                              3 marks
- Basophilic stippling.
- Inclusion bodies.
- Microcytosis.
- Hypochromic red cells.

c.   Blood transfusions.                                      1 mark

d.   Any 4 from:                                              2 marks
- Joint pain.
- Erectile dysfunction.
- Abdominal pain.
- Skin bronzing.
- Hair loss.
- Depression.
- Fatigue.

e.   Desferrioxamine.                                         2 marks

**10)**

a. Autogenic: stem cells belonging to the patient.    2 marks
Allogenic: stem cells belonging to a genetically similar but not identical donor.

b. Barrier precautions.    2 marks
Secure central venous access.

c. Any 2 from:    2 marks
- Susceptibility to infection.
- Graft failure.
- Graft versus host disease.
- Pain.
- Thrombocytopenia.
- Circulatory overload.
- Reactivation of latent infections.
- Immunosuppression.

d. Donor cells attack the recipient's cells.    3 marks
Any 2 from:
- Skin.
- Liver.
- Eyes.
- Lung.
- Gut.

e. Type 4 hypersensitivity.    1 mark

**11)**

a. A bridge glycoprotein (1 mark), two binding sites: factor VIII and platelets (1 mark) and ensures platelets are bound to exposed endothelium (1 mark).    3 marks

b. Autosomal dominant.    1 mark

c. Low levels of von Willebrand's factor in blood.    2 marks
Defective von Willebrand's factor.

d. Haemophilia (A or B).    2 marks

e. X-linked recessive.    2 marks

12)

a. Polycythaemia rubra vera (PRV).                                    2 marks

b. JAK 2 mutation.                                                    2 marks

c. Any 2 from:                                                        2 marks

- Smoking.
- Altitude.
- Cyanotic congenital heart disease.
- COPD.
- EPO-secreting tumour.

d. Venesection.                                                      1 mark

e. Any 2 from:                                                        3 marks

- Hypertension.
- Stroke.
- Thromboses.
- Peripheral vascular disease.
- Ischaemic heart disease.

At risk of acute lymphoblastic leukaemia (1 mark).

13)

a. A-E assessment.                                                   1 mark

b. Any 4 from:                                                        2 marks

- Peripheral blood cultures.
- Line blood cultures.
- ABG.
- Chest X-ray.
- Sputum MC&S.
- Urine MC&S.

c. Broad-spectrum antibiotics.                                      2 marks

d. Viral reactivation.                                              3 marks

Bacterial.

Fungal.

e. *Pneumocystis carinii*.                                         2 marks

# Chapter 17

# Rheumatology

## ANSWERS

1) c.
2) b.
3) a.
4) a.
5) d.
6) b.
7) b.
8) c.
9) d.
10) a.
11) a.
12) c.
13) d.
14) a.
15) a.
16) b.
17) c.
18) d.
19) a.
20) c.

21) d.
22) b.
23) d.

# Extended matching question answers

1) c

Weakness on walking up stairs and raising the arms above the head is classic of a proximal muscle weakness. The papules described are Gottron's papules which distinguishes this from polymyositis.

2) e

The phenomenon being described is Raynaud's phenomenon, but with the history of gastric reflux (oesophageal dysmotility) and telangiectasia, CREST syndrome should be considered.

3) b

Isoniazid is known to precipitate drug-induced lupus, which resolves on stopping the drug. Other common causes include hydralazine and procainamide.

4) f

Symptoms can be explained by Sjögren syndrome; dry eyes, dry mouth (causing problems swallowing) and vaginal dryness.

5) b

Amlodipine is known to cause drug-induced lupus.

6) e

The age and the fact that the pain gets worse on activity points to osteoarthritis.

7) h

Gout can affect the knee joint with a sudden onset of pain. There is no history of trauma or activity making prepatellar bursitis less likely.

8) g

DIP involvement is rare in early rheumatoid arthritis making psoriatic arthritis more likely. Arthritis can precede the characteristic rash in psoriatic arthritis by several years.

9) d

A group A streptococcal URTI can cause reactive arthritis. Osgood-Schlatter disease would be worse with activity. Bursitis would present acutely.

10) c

Rheumatoid arthritis is more common than psoriatic arthritis, although both can cause the pattern of joint involvement described.

11) g

This is a classic description of erythema nodosum. It is seen in Sjögren syndrome.

12) d

Gouty tophi are pathognomonic. A rheumatoid nodule would not have a chalky appearance.

13) b

Keratoderma blennorrhagica is commonly seen in reactive arthritis.

14) c

20-30% of patients with rheumatoid arthritis develop rheumatoid nodules.

15) a

Pyoderma gangrenosum is a complication of rheumatoid arthritis.

16) a

Colchicine is often limited by its gastrointestinal side effects.

17) d

Patients should be warned of blood disorders (e.g. easy bruising, sore throat, mouth ulcers), liver toxicity and respiratory symptoms before starting methotrexate. Whilst other rheumatological drugs can cause myelosuppression, this is the first-line treatment and therefore the most likely drug this female would be taking.

18) f

Patients commencing TNF-alpha blockers should be screened for active or latent TB due to the risk of reactivation.

19) h

Corticosteroids cause altered glucose metabolism, which can in turn lead to poor healing and other complications.

20) b

NSAIDs can cause gastric ulcers. A PPI should be co-prescribed with long-term use.

21) b

This is more common in people of Asian descent. It is a large-vessel vasculitis mainly affecting the aorta and its main branches. The hypertension is due to renal artery stenosis.

22) h

Other features of the disease include iritis and skin lesions. It is due to an immune-mediated occlusive vasculitis.

23) e

This is also known as Wegener's granulomatosis, a vasculitis of small- and medium-sized vessels, often presenting with 'ELK' symptoms (ear, lungs, kidney). Patients may have a saddle-shaped nose.

24) a

This is a classic description of Henoch-Schönlein purpura (HSP), a small-vessel vasculitis. The third symptom in the classic triad is abdominal pain.

25) g

He may also complain of jaw claudication. It is associated with polymyalgia rheumatica.

26) g

Anti-nuclear antibody (ANA) is found in >95% of patients with SLE but is not specific. Anti-dsDNA is more specific but less sensitive.

27) b

Seen in Sjögren syndrome, neonatal lupus and ANA-negative SLE.

28) a

c-ANCA is associated with Wegener's granulomatosis. p-ANCA is associated with Churg-Strauss syndrome.

29) c

Anti-glomerular basement membrane antibodies attack Type IV collagen in the kidneys and lungs in Goodpasture's syndrome.

30) d

This is found in 80-90% of patients with CREST syndrome (limited scleroderma with systemic involvement).

31) e

This lady has fibromyalgia; widespread body pain lasting >3 months, often associated with poor sleep. There are no systemic features described, making this more likely than the other options.

32) b

Polymyositis affects proximal muscles (problems climbing stairs, raising arms above head) with systemic features (fever, weight loss, malaise). No rash is mentioned in the history, excluding dermatomyositis. Polymyalgia rheumatica tends to affect patients over 50, and lower limb weakness is not a feature.

33) g

SLE can present with a wide range of symptoms, which may be non-specific. The rash described points to SLE (malar rash) and is not typical of dermatomyositis.

34) a

He may also complain of flu-like symptoms. The condition is associated with giant cell arteritis.

35) f

Symptoms need to have lasted for >6 months with at least four of the diagnostic criteria (headache, joint pains without swelling/erythema, muscular pain, exertional malaise, impaired concentration, sore throat, unrefreshing sleep, tender lymph nodes). It is often triggered by an illness or a stressful event. The main complaint of this lady is fatigue, whereas in fibromyalgia it is pain.

36) e

Skin lesions seen in SLE respond well to hydroxychloroquine.

37) a

Physiotherapy is used in conjunction with NSAIDs.

38) f

Methotrexate is the most commonly used first-line DMARD in rheumatoid arthritis.

39) b

Other calcium channel blockers are not licensed for the treatment of Raynaud's disease.

40) c

Visual symptoms in GCA require admission and treatment with IV methylprednisolone to prevent visual loss. Oral prednisolone would be used if eye symptoms were not present.

41) c

Aortic regurgitation is a complication of ankylosing spondylitis. The description of the murmur does not correlate with any of the other options.

42) h

Widespread ST elevation and sharp chest pain points to a diagnosis of pericarditis as opposed to MI.

43) b

The vegetations in Libman-Sacks endocarditis are formed from inflammatory cells and fibrin.

44) g

Pulmonary hypertension is often a consequence of interstitial lung disease in systemic sclerosis.

45) e

Coronary artery aneurysms usually develop within 10 days of onset of illness. It predisposes to an MI.

# Short answer question answers

1)

a. Any 2 from: 2 marks
- ANA.
- Anti-dsDNA.
- Anti-SM.
- Anti-Ro.
- Anti-La.
- Anti-histone.

b. Any 6 from: 3 marks
- Fever.
- Malaise.
- Lymphadenopathy.
- Weight loss.
- Oral ulcers.
- Pleuritic chest pain.
- Paraesthesia.
- Dry eyes and mouth.
- Raynaud's phenomenon.
- Hair loss.
- Myalgia.
- Joint swelling.
- Anxiety.
- Depression.

c. Sun cream. 1 mark

d. Hydroxychloroquine. 2 marks

e. Libman-Sacks endocarditis. 2 marks

2)

a.  Any 2 from:                                              2 marks
    - Tongue claudication.
    - Jaw claudication.
    - Visual symptoms.

b.  Any 3 from:                                              3 marks
    - Tender temporal artery.
    - Thickened temporal artery.
    - Beaded temporal artery.
    - Reduced/absent pulsation of temporal artery.
    - Scalp tenderness.
    - Reduced visual acuity.
    - Visual field defect.
    - Afferent pupillary defect.
    - Pale/swollen optic disc.
    - Retinal artery occlusion.
    - Carotid bruits.
    - Pyrexia.

c.  Raised ESR.                                              1 mark

d.  Temporal artery biopsy.                                  2 marks

e.  High-dose corticosteroids.                               2 marks
    Aspirin.

3)

a.  Anti-CCP.                                                2 marks

b.  Any 4 from:                                              4 marks
    - Ulnar deviation of MCP joints.
    - Boutonnière deformity of the fingers.
    - Swan-neck deformity of the fingers.
    - Z-deformity of the thumb.
    - MCP subluxation.
    - Muscle wasting.

c.  Methotrexate.                                                         1 mark

d.  Folic acid (methotrexate inhibits folate metabolism).                1 mark

e.  Normocytic normochromic anaemia.                                     2 marks

4)

a.  Gottron's papules.                                                   1 mark

b.  Any 2 from:                                                          2 marks
    - Heliotrope discoloration of eyelids.
    - Periorbital oedema.
    - Dilated capillary loops under the fingernails.
    - Erythematous macules.

c.  Creatinine kinase.                                                   2 marks

d.  Any 3 from:                                                          3 marks
    - Muscle swelling.
    - Muscle tenderness.
    - Arthralgia.
    - Fatigue.
    - Dysphagia (pharyngeal weakness).
    - Fever.
    - Muscle cramps.
    - Raynaud's phenomenon.
    - Mouth ulcers.

e.  Corticosteroids.                                                     2 marks

5)

a.  Any 4 from:                                                          4 marks
    - Sleep disturbance.
    - Morning stiffness.
    - Paraesthesia.
    - Feeling of swollen joints (with no objective evidence).
    - Memory disturbance.
    - Difficulty concentrating.
    - Headache.

- Light-headedness.
- Dizziness.

b. Any 2 from:          1 mark
- Supervised exercise therapy.
- CBT.
- Physiotherapy.
- Psychological support.

c. Antidepressants.          1 mark

d. Any 3 from:          3 marks
- Primary care doctor.
- Rheumatologist.
- Chronic pain physician.
- Psychiatrist.
- Physiotherapist.

e. Any 2 from:          1 mark
- Female sex.
- Age between 20-50 years.
- Past medical history of anxiety and depression.
- Separation with partner.

6)

a. Urethritis.          1 mark

b. Any 1 from:          1 mark
- Mouth ulcers.
- Erythema nodosum.
- Circinate balanitis.
- Keratoderma blennorrhagica.

c. Any 4 from:          4 marks
- *Yersinia spp.*
- *Salmonella spp.*
- *Shigella spp.*
- *Campylobacter spp.*
- *Clostridium difficile.*
- *E. coli O157.*

d. Any 1 from:     2 marks
- Pericarditis.
- Aortitis.
- Aortic regurgitation.
- Conduction defects.

e. Complete resolution.     2 marks

7)

a. Any 3 from:     3 marks
- Dactylitis.
- Nail pitting.
- Onycholysis.
- Nail discolouration.
- Subungual hyperkeratosis.

b. Any 3 from:     3 marks
- Periosteal new bone formation.
- Soft tissue swelling.
- Bony erosions.
- 'Pencil in cup' deformity.
- Loss of joint space.
- Joint subluxation.

c. Arthritis mutilans.     1 mark

d. Any 2 from:     2 marks
- Leflunomide.
- Sulfasalazine.
- Methotrexate.
- Ciclosporin.

e. Anti-TNFa therapy.     1 mark

8)

a. HLA B27.     1 mark

b.  Any 4 from:           4 marks
- Anterior uveitis.
- Aortic incompetence.
- Apical lung fibrosis.
- Aortitis.
- Amyloidosis.
- Heart block.

c.  Physiotherapy.           2 marks
    NSAIDs.

d.  Any 2 from:           2 marks
- Sacroiliitis (subchondral erosion, sclerosis, fusion).
- Loss of lumbar lordosis.
- Squaring of vertebrae.
- Bamboo spine (calcification of spinal ligament).

e.  Cauda equina syndrome.           1 mark


9)

a.  Any 6 from:           3 marks
- Fatigue.
- Malaise.
- Weakness.
- Anorexia.
- Weight loss.
- Wheeze.
- Facial pain.
- Cough.
- Shortness of breath.
- Chest pain.
- Joint pain.
- Abdominal pain.
- Hearing loss.
- Nasal ulcers.
- Rashes.

- Haematuria.
- Chronic ear infections.
- Rhinorrhoea.

b. Subglottic stenosis. 2 marks

c. Any 2 from: 2 marks
- Ulcers and crusting around the nose.
- Destruction of nasal cartilage.
- Rhinorrhoea.
- Conjunctivitis.
- Scleritis.
- Episcleritis.

d. ANCA. 1 mark

e. Cyclophosphamide. 2 marks

## 10)

a. Negatively birefringent needle-shaped crystals. 2 marks

b. Hyperuricaemia. 2 marks

c. Any 1 from: 1 mark
- NSAIDs.
- Colchicine.
- Prednisolone.

d. Gouty tophus. 2 marks

e. Any 3 from: 3 marks
- Lose weight.
- Reduce alcohol intake.
- Keep well hydrated.
- Consume a low purine diet.
- Ensure good diabetic control.

## 11)

a. HLA DR4. 2 marks
HLA DR1.

b.     Carpal tunnel syndrome.                                          2 marks
c.     Any 1 from:                                                      2 marks
       ● Age of onset <30 years.
       ● Insidious onset.
d.     DAS28.                                                           2 marks
e.     Any 1 from:                                                      2 marks
       ● Adalimumab.
       ● Etanercept.
       ● Infliximab.
       ● Certolizumab pegol.


12)
a.     Joint aspiration.                                                2 marks
b.     Calcium pyrophosphate.                                           2 marks
c.     Any 3 from:                                                      3 marks
       ● Dehydration.
       ● Hyperparathyroidism.
       ● Corticosteroids.
       ● Hypothyroidism.
       ● Haemochromatosis.
       ● Wilson's disease.
       ● Acromegaly.
       ● Dialysis.
       ● Surgery.
       ● Trauma.
       ● Hypomagnesaemia.
d.     Linear opacification of the articular cartilage.                 2 marks
e.     Usually resolves within 10 days.                                 1 mark

13)

a. Eosinophilia >10% in the peripheral blood. 2 marks

b. Any 2 from: 2 marks
- Anaemia.
- Elevated ESR.
- Elevated CRP.
- Elevated creatinine.
- Elevated IgE.

c. ANCA. 1 mark

d. Any 4 from: 4 marks
- Heart failure.
- Myocarditis.
- Glomerulonephritis.
- Hypertension.
- Stroke.
- Bowel ischaemia.
- Bowel perforation.
- Pancreatitis.
- Appendicitis.
- Renal failure.
- Digital ischaemia.

e. High-dose corticosteroids. 1 mark

# Chapter 18

# Infectious disease

## ANSWERS

1) c.
2) d.
3) c.
4) a.
5) a.
6) b.
7) c.
8) d.
9) b.
10) a.
11) b.
12) c.
13) c.
14) d.
15) b.
16) d.
17) a.
18) b.
19) a.
20) c.

21) a.
22) c.
23) d.

# Extended matching question answers

1) a

Turbid CSF with a high proportion of polymorphonuclear leukocytes is usually indicative of bacterial meningitis.

2) c

Clear CSF with normal/mildly raised WBCs, mildly elevated protein and an oligoclonal band on electrophoresis is consistent with MS. The glucose CSF level in MS should be normal.

3) e

In viral meningitis, CSF is usually clear with an elevated WBC count predominantly formed of lymphocytes, a normal glucose and mildly elevated protein level.

4) d

A lumbar puncture in idiopathic intracranial hypertension is unremarkable, other than a raised opening pressure.

5) h

You may also see a high WBC count in tuberculous meningitis but this is typically lymphocyte predominant. Other signs of TB include fibrin web formation and a very high protein >1.5g/L.

6) f

*Bacillus cereus* is a Gram-positive bacillus and typically infects contaminated rice and produces two toxins leading to vomiting or diarrhoea. Vomiting usually occurs 2-5 hours after ingestion and diarrhoea 12 hours after ingestion. It usually last for 12-24 hours.

7)   a

The classical description of symptoms for *Vibrio cholera* are described in this question. It is transmitted in a faecal oral route and there is a spectrum of symptoms from mild diarrhoea to severe dehydration. The classical stool description is rice water.

8)   b

*E. coli O517* causes a diarrhoeal illness that can lead to haemolytic uraemic syndrome, as in this question. Contact with farm animals is a common route of transmission. Rotavirus is another cause of gastroenteritis in children. It can spread quickly around nurseries; however, it is usually self-limiting and conservatively managed.

9)   h

*Campylobacter jejuni* is a known risk factor for the development of Guillain-Barré syndrome.

10)  g

*Staphylococcus aureus* leads to a rapid onset of symptoms due to the presence of a pre-formed toxin. Symptoms are usually self-limiting and occur following ingestion of contaminated food. Treatment is supportive using fluid management.

11)  d

A flu-like illness and jaundice could be a presentation of any of the above. The clue is the patient's occupation which puts him at risk of exposure to urine of infected animals; therefore, leptospirosis is the correct answer. The jaundice and acute kidney injury are typical of Weil's disease.

12)  e

This is classic of Epstein-Barr virus presenting as glandular fever. *Cytomegalovirus* may present similarly; however, it is more likely to present in an immunocompromised patient without pharyngitis and lymphadenopathy.

13) g

Thick and thin blood smears are used to diagnose malaria.

14) c

Both hepatitis B and hepatitis C can present acutely and lead to chronic hepatitis. Hepatitis C is much more likely to lead to chronic infection than hepatitis B which more typically presents acutely. They are both transmitted by the same routes. Blood tests for antigens and antibodies are required to differentiate between them. Hepatitis C increases the risk of certain extra-hepatic diseases including autoimmune conditions such as Sjögren's syndrome.

15) a

Hepatitis A is faecal-orally transmitted. There is usually a history of recent foreign travel associated with a mild flu-like illness, anorexia and jaundice. Shellfish may have been eaten recently and other clues include a sudden distaste for cigarette smoking.

16) f

*Pseudomonas aeruginosa* is seen in patients with immunosuppression and chronic lung diseases such as cystic fibrosis and bronchiectasis.

17) h

*Chlamydophila psittaci* is a pneumonia normally related to exposure to birds that may be unwell.

18) a

*Streptococcus pneumoniae* is the most common cause of community-acquired pneumonia.

19)   c

Mycoplasma pneumoniae may present over weeks. The cough is often dry and has many extra-respiratory manifestations including erythema multiforme (target lesions) and haemolytic anaemia.

20)   d

Staphylococcus aureus pneumonia often occurs following influenza or other viral infections such as measles.

21)   b

Measles presents with a rash and classically with a cough, coryza and conjunctivitis. Koplik spots are found on the buccal mucosa and are red spots with a speck in the centre; these are pathognomonic of measles. Rubella is a viral exanthem that may be difficult to differentiate from measles; the pink macular rash typically develops behind the ears and spreads downwards.

22)   c

Epiglottitis is a medical emergency and presents as described. In suspected epiglottitis, the throat should not be examined due to the risk of inducing laryngeal obstruction. Differentiating between croup and epiglottitis may be difficult. Children with croup tend to be well looking, have a barking cough and are able to swallow their own secretions. Croup is most commonly caused by the parainfluenza virus and in more severe cases, children may have respiratory distress and stridor.

23)   g

Scarlet fever has a rash with a coarse sandpaper-like texture. They may also have a strawberry tongue and pharyngitis on examination, caused by a Group A streptococcal infection.

24) a

Whooping cough is usually caused by *Bordetella pertussis*, characterised by a severe cough which may be followed by a 'whoop' sound. Post-cough vomiting is common and the cough can persist for months.

25) h

Children with croup tend to be well looking, have a barking cough and are able to swallow their own secretions. Croup is most commonly caused by the parainfluenza virus and in more severe cases, children may have respiratory distress and stridor.

26) d

Vancomycin is a glycopeptide that is useful in managing MRSA bacteraemia and *Clostridium difficile* infection.

27) f

Ceftriaxone is a third-generation cephalosporin useful in meningitis. It should not be used in patients who are anaphylactic to penicillin as there is cross-reactivity between them.

28) c

Metronidazole is effective against anaerobes. Patients are advised not to consume alcohol as they can experience unpleasant effects, usually severe nausea and vomiting.

29) e

Clarithromycin is a macrolide antibiotic recommended alongside co-amoxiclav; it is effective against atypical pneumonias.

30) g

Ciprofloxacin is a fluoroquinolone with many uses. It should be avoided in patients with epilepsy. It has good Gram-negative cover and can be used in intra-abdominal infections. It is known to reduce the seizure threshold; therefore, it is contraindicated in epilepsy.

31)  d

*Cryptococcus* meningitis is found in immunosuppressed individuals and Indian ink stain aids diagnosis.

32)  a

Listeria is associated with soft cheese. It is resistant to cephalosporins typically given such as ceftriaxone; therefore, in suspected cases of listeria meningitis, ampicillin is added to cover for it. It is usually found in the elderly or the immunocompromised.

33)  b

*Neisseria meningitidis* is the most common cause of meningitis in children and young adults. It is a Gram-negative diplococcus.

34)  f

Group B *Streptococcus* is often found asymptomatically in the vagina and birth canal. It is not routinely screened for in the UK. Typical presentations of Group B *Streptococcus* in a newborn include septicaemia without an obvious cause, pneumonia and meningitis.

35)  e

A brain abscess can occur as a result of localised or remote spread. It is more common in immunosuppressed patients. On questioning, the patient will classically mention a recent dental abscess or sinus infection. There is a triad of fever, headache and focal neurology. A CT of the head with a brain abscess typically shows a solitary ring-enhancing lesion.

36) c

Trichomonas vaginalis is a flagellated protozoan. It commonly presents with frothy greenish vaginal discharge and itching. A strawberry cervix may be found on examination. It is treated with metronidazole.

37) f

Gonorrhoea is caused by a Gram-negative diplococcus (*Neisseria gonorrhoeae*) and usually presents with purulent urethritis. Due to emerging resistance it is treated with ceftriaxone and azithromycin.

38) a

Bacterial vaginosis often presents with whitish-grey vaginal discharge with a fishy smell, most commonly caused by *Gardnerella vaginalis*. The clue cells are found on microscopy and it is treated with metronidazole.

39) b

*Chlamydia trachomatis* is an intracellular Gram-negative bacteria that is commonly asymptomatic and is detected on routine screening. It is the most commonly diagnosed sexually transmitted infection in the UK and untreated can significantly impact fertility.

40) d

Genital warts are benign lesions caused by the human papilloma virus. They are usually painless. The incidence of genital warts alongside cervical cancer has been reduced in several countries after the implementation of HPV vaccination programmes.

41) f

*Cytomegalovirus* retinitis presents with visual disturbance, often of the central vision and has pizza pie changes on fundoscopy.

42) d

Cytomegalovirus infection can also cause diarrhoea; however, it typically causes other symptoms such as abdominal pain or fever; therefore, Cryptosporidium is the most likely cause.

43) e

Oesophageal candidiasis causes painful swallowing as it is caused by Candida albicans. It responds to antifungal therapy such as fluconazole.

44) a

Kaposi's sarcoma is caused by the human Herpes virus 8. It presents typically in HIV as raised purplish-red lesions often around the mouth that can coalesce to form plaques and may rapidly increase in size. Women with HIV are at a higher risk of developing cervical cancer. It is caused by certain strains of the human papilloma virus.

45) c

Pneumocystis jirovecii presents with symptoms of pneumonia. There may be little in the way of chest signs or X-ray changes. The classical examination finding is desaturation on exertion. It is usually treated with co-trimoxazole.

# Short answer question answers

**1)**

a. Any 2 from:      2 marks
- *Streptococcus pneumoniae.*
- *Haemophilus influenzae.*
- *Staphylococcus aureus.*
- *Klebsiella pneumoniae.*
- *Mycoplasma pneumoniae.*
- *Legionella pneumophila.*
- *Chlamydophila pneumoniae.*

b. Any 3 from:      3 marks
- Chest X-ray.
- Sputum culture.
- ABG.
- Urinary antigens.

c. CURB-65 score.      1 mark

d. A penicillin-based antibiotic, e.g. co-amoxiclav.      2 marks
A macrolide antibiotic, e.g. clarithromycin, erythromycin.

e. Any 2 from:      2 marks
- Pleurisy.
- Pleural effusion (parapneumonic).
- Empyema.
- Lung abscess.
- Pneumothorax.
- Acute kidney injury.
- Sepsis.
- Bronchiectasis.

2)

a. Any 2 from:      2 marks
- Palpable notch on the anterior border of the spleen.
- Kidney is ballotable; the spleen is not.
- Unable to palpate the upper edge of the spleen which you are able to do with the kidney.

b. Monospot test.      2 marks

c. Atypical lymphocytes.      2 marks

d. Any 3 from:      3 marks
- *Cytomegalovirus*.
- Viral hepatitis.
- Human immunodeficiency virus.
- Toxoplasmosis.
- Rubella.
- Mumps.
- Roseola.

e. Avoid contact sports for 4 weeks.      1 mark

3)

a. Type 1 respiratory failure.      2 marks
    Hypoxia.

b. *Pneumocystis jirovecii*.      2 marks

c. Any 4 from:      4 marks
- Oesophageal candidiasis.
- Pulmonary candidiasis.
- Cervical cancer.
- Non-Hodgkin's lymphoma.
- *Cytomegalovirus* retinitis.
- HIV-related encephalopathy.
- Kaposi's sarcoma.
- *Mycobacterium avium* complex.
- *Mycobacterium tuberculosis*.
- Cerebral toxoplasmosis.
- Recurrent pneumonia.

d.   Co-trimoxazole.                                    1 mark
e.   CD4 count.                                         1 mark

4)
a.   *Entamoeba histolytica*.                           2 marks
b.   Liver abscess.                                     2 marks
c.   Any four rows from Table 18.1.                     4 marks

## Table 18.1

| Test | Example of satisfactory reason |
| --- | --- |
| Full blood count (FBC) | Patient pale, may be anaemic, may have a raised WCC |
| Inflammatory markers (e.g. CRP, ESR) | Patient has a fever, likely to be raised; if not raised, consider another diagnosis |
| Serology | Diagnostic confirmation |
| Blood cultures | Patient pyrexial, may have a bacteraemia |
| Liver function tests (LFTs) | Hepatomegaly on examination |
| Urea & electrolytes (U&Es) | Insensible losses from fever, poor oral intake, may require IV fluids |
| Group and save | Previously bloody diarrhoea and looks pale, may possibly require a blood transfusion |
| Glucose | May be low due to reduced oral intake |

d.  Ultrasound scan of the abdomen.                                    1 mark

e.  Any 1 from:                                                         1 mark

- Good personal hygiene with hand washing.
- Drink bottled water.
- Adequate sanitation.

5)

a.  Thick and thin blood films.                                        2 marks

b.  *Plasmodium vivax* enters a dormant stage as liver hypnozoites.    3 marks
    Hypnozoites do not occur in *Plasmodium falciparum* infection.
    These can reactivate and lead to relapse.

c.  Glucose-6-phosphate dehydrogenase deficiency.                      1 mark

d.  Any 2 from:                                                        2 marks

- Take anti-malarial prophylaxis/chemoprophylaxis.
- Use insecticide treated nets.
- Avoid outdoor activity after sunset.
- Wear long-sleeved shirts and trousers.
- Use insect repellent.

e.  Any 2 from:                                                        2 marks

- Acute infectious hepatitis.
- Acute meningitis.
- Cholera.
- Diphtheria.
- Typhoid fever.
- Food poisoning.
- Haemolytic uraemic syndrome.
- Legionnaires' disease.
- Measles.
- Mumps.
- Rabies.
- Rubella.
- Scarlet fever.
- Tetanus.

- Tuberculosis.
- Viral haemorrhagic fever.
- Whooping cough.

6)

a. Benzylpenicillin.                                     2 marks
   Intra-muscular.
b. Eye opening.                                          3 marks
   Verbal response.
   Motor response.
c. Blood cultures.                                       3 marks
   Accurate urine output measurement.
   IV fluids.
   Antibiotics.
   Lactate.
   Oxygen.
d. *Neisseria meningitidis*.                             1 mark
e. Any 1 from:                                           1 mark
   - Ciprofloxacin.
   - Rifampicin.

7)

a. Any 2 from:                                           2 marks
   - Sexual intercourse.
   - Intravenous drug use.
   - Blood transfusion.
   - Vertical transmission.
   - Pregnancy.
   - Needle stick injury.
   - Use of unsterile equipment.
b. Any 8 from:                                           4 marks
   - LFTs.
   - Clotting.
   - FBC.

- U&Es.
- Viral hepatitis serology.
- Ferritin.
- Iron studies.
- Alpha-1 antitrypsin.
- Immunoglobulins.
- Protein electrophoresis.
- Autoantibodies.
- α-fetoprotein.
- Serum copper.
- Caeruloplasmin.
- Lipid profile.

c. Ultrasound abdomen.    1 mark

d. Any 2 from:    2 marks
- Bilirubin.
- Albumin.
- Prothrombin time.
- Ascites.
- Hepatic encephalopathy.

e. To stop drinking alcohol.    1 mark

8)

a. *Staphylococcus aureus*.    1 mark

b. Any 3 from:    3 marks
- Gout.
- Pseudogout.
- Reactive arthritis.
- Rheumatoid arthritis.
- Osteoarthritis.
- Haemarthrosis.
- Trauma.

c. Joint aspiration.    1 mark

d.     i. Gout: negatively birefringent needles.       4 marks

        ii. Pseudogout: positively birefringent rhomboid-shaped crystals.

e.     HbA1c.        1 mark

## 9)

a.     Any 4 from:        4 marks

- Reduced skin turgor.
- Prolonged capillary refill.
- Sunken eyes.
- Impaired level of consciousness.
- Dry mucous membranes.
- Tachycardia.
- Hypotension.
- Reduced JVP.

b.     Cholera.        1 mark

c.     Metabolic acidosis with partial respiratory compensation.        2 marks

d.     *Escherichia coli*.        1 mark

e.     Any 2 from:        2 marks

- Drink bottled water.
- Peel fruit and vegetables.
- Avoid ice.
- Avoid shellfish.
- Cook food thoroughly.
- Hand hygiene.

## 10)

a.     Any 4 from:        4 marks

- Patient's age.
- Prolonged hospital stay.
- Multiple courses of antibiotics.
- Use of proton pump inhibitor.
- Multiple comorbidities.
- Current symptoms (fever and loose stools).
- Foul-smelling stools.

| | | |
|---|---|---|
| b. | Bristol Stool Chart. | 1 mark |
| c. | Metronidazole. | 1 mark |
| d. | Oral vancomycin. | 2 marks |
| e. | Any 2 from: | 2 marks |

- Isolate the patient in a side room.
- Barrier nursing.
- Strict hand hygiene.
- Use of gloves and aprons.

11)

a. Any 2 from:      2 marks

- Social overcrowding.
- Close contact with a TB patient.
- Intravenous drug use.
- HIV.
- Immunocompromised patient.

b. i. Peripheral neuropathy — isoniazid.      4 marks
   ii. Red/orange urine — rifampicin.
   iii. Optic neuritis — ethambutol.
   iv. Gout — pyrazinamide.

c. Directly observed treatment.      1 mark

d. Any 1 from:      1 mark

- Mantoux test.
- Interferon gamma testing.

e. Caseating granulomas.      2 marks

12)

a. Any 4 from:      4 marks

- Purulent vaginal discharge.
- Increased amount of vaginal discharge.
- Lower abdominal pain.
- Deep dyspareunia.
- Fever.
- Dysuria.

- Intermenstrual bleeding.
- Postcoital bleeding.
- Urinary frequency.

b. Any 2 from:     2 marks
  - Cervical excitation.
  - Adnexal tenderness.
  - Abdominal tenderness.
  - Mucopurulent cervical discharge.
  - Inflamed cervix that may bleed when touched.

c. Nucleic acid amplification tests.     1 mark

d. Any 1 from:     1 mark
  - Doxycycline.
  - Azithromycin.

e. Any 2 from:     2 marks
  - Pelvic inflammatory disease.
  - Subfertility or infertility.
  - Ectopic pregnancy.
  - Reactive arthritis.
  - Fitz-Hugh-Curtis syndrome.
  - Chronic pelvic pain.

13)

a. *Varicella zoster* virus.     2 marks

b. *Varicella zoster* lies dormant in sensory ganglia of nerve cells   2 marks
following primary infection (1 mark). A decrease in cell-mediated
immunity leads to virus reactivation (1 mark).

c. i. As she works as a school teacher and the lesions are weeping, she   2 marks
should not go to work.

   ii. She is no longer infectious when all the lesions have crusted over.

d. i. Post-herpetic neuralgia.     3 marks

   ii. Any 2 from:
  - Amitriptyline.
  - Pregabalin.

- Gabapentin.
- Duloxetine.

e.    Ramsay Hunt syndrome.                                    1 mark

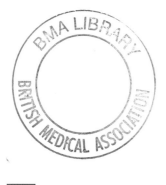